ADVENTURES IN

DIET LAND

Marci x Rob,
for Everything!

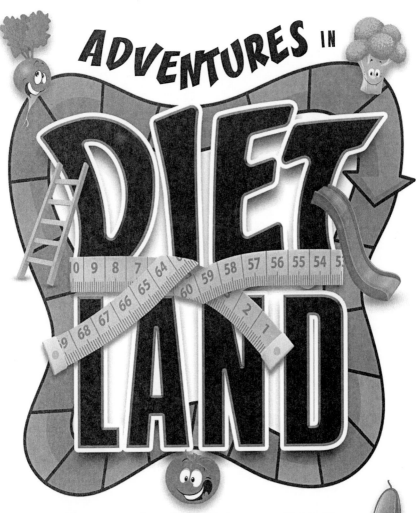

ADVENTURES IN DIET LAND

How to Win at the Game of Dieting
from a **FORMER FAT GUY**

RALPH PETERSON

9 8 7 6 5 4 3 2 1

Digit on the right indicates the number of this printing

ISBN: 978-0-9989268-0-3

Cover and interior design by Jerry Dorris (www.authorsupport.com)

Back of the book picture by Sandy Sarza

Editorial support by Author Bridge Media

Legal Disclaimer

I am not your doctor. In fact, I am no one's doctor. I haven't stepped one foot into a medical school. Well, that's not true. I think I may have walked around Dartmouth once, but that was strictly as a visitor, and in no way makes me qualified to tell you what you should be eating, or shouldn't be eating, or what you should be doing, or how you should be living your life.

Please contact your nearest medical professional before starting any diets, or making any changes to your diets, beginning a new workout routine, or if you feel pain anywhere. -Seriously, go see your doctor.

Further, I am not an expert on diets. I think I can safely say that I have tried most of them, and have a pretty good understanding as to why some things worked for me and why others didn't. However, that is not a reflection of the diet plans themselves, as much as it was my own inability to follow them.

Full disclosure, I follow the Weight Watchers Diet Plan. It, along with the "**50 Rules Everyone Needs to Know, to Win at the Game of Dieting**" found in this book, works for me. However, I am not associated with Weight Watchers in any way. I should be. But I'm not. As far as I can tell, they have no idea who I am. Yet.

Finally, I do believe most diet plans have merit and can work if you apply them. You just have to find the one that works for you. No diet plans were harmed in the writing of this book.

Best of luck,
Ralph

This book is dedicated to everyone who, like me, continues to push back against the voice in our heads. That constant voice who whispers it is too hard... we are too weak and unmotivated. We lack skills and focus. The voice that tries to convince us we cannot change our destiny, we were born this way... uneducated, unworthy... Fat.

The voice is wrong. Continue to fight.

It's worth it. YOU are worth it.

Table of Contents

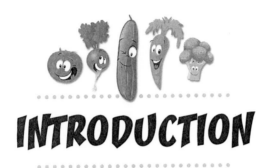

INTRODUCTION

"What, are you eating," I said when I walked into Adams office. He had a large stack of bologna, a stack of cheese and a jar of mayonnaise, open, with a knife sticking out of it, on his desk. He looked up with the biggest grin on his face.

"What," he said. "I'm on Atkins."

"Oh, Adam." I said shaking my head and putting my bag down. "You're doing it all wrong."

"No I'm not," he said. "I can eat as much of this as I want.

Bologna and cheese doesn't have any carbs… and neither does mayonnaise." Adam has one of the most infectious grins and when he smiles, you cannot help but smile back. Then I got all scientific on him, because I'm that asshole.

"I'll give you the bologna and mayonnaise, because they definitely don't have carbs, but you have to be careful with cheese because it does have some."

"Yeah, but not enough to make a real difference," Adam said. I shrugged.

"It depends on where you are with Atkins," I said. "If you are doing the Induction Phase, then you really need to limit your carb intake to single digits, like really, really low or you will never get into a state of ketosis. Which is the whole point of the Induction phase."

"That reminds me," Adam said. "I need to buy some of those strips that you pee on."

"Ketostix Strips," I said. While we were talking one of Adam's assistants (Nate) poked his head into the office, smiled at us but stayed outside. I called him in.

"You don't have to wait out there," I said. "We're just talking about Adam's eating habits." He came in smiling.

"What do you think of Adam's diet," he said gesturing to the bologna, cheese and mayonnaise on his desk.

"You're just jealous," Adam said. We all laughed and then Nate asked me what everyone asks me. Everyone who knew me from before.

"Did you do Atkins?" I nodded.

"A bunch of times," I said, "but I never had any success with it. To be honest, I always ended up gaining more weight than I lost with Atkins." I looked at Adam. Then at his stomach. Then back at Adam. Then back at his stomach.

"What," he said laughing and trying to cover it up. "Don't you look over here Mr. Peterson." We all laughed. Then we jumped down the dieter's rabbit hole and started discussing all the diets I've tried and what worked and what didn't.

"I'm telling you. You should write a book," Adam said. "About all of the diets you've tried." I laughed, not sure if I liked the idea or not.

"I'm serious," he said. "I would buy that book. Everyone wants to know how you lost all your weight..."

"How much have you lost," Nate said.

"Around 150 pounds," I said. Nate whistled.

"Wow," he said dragging out the word. I nodded and smiled. I love seeing people's reactions. Adam spoke up.

"And the best part is you didn't cheat." I looked at him furrowing my eyebrows.

"Cheat?"

"Yeah. You know. You didn't have surgery or do something stupid like stop eating for forty days."

"True," I said.

"Of course, there was something about a coffee enema," he said. I could feel my face start to turn red.

"That had nothing to do with dieting," I said.

"But you don't deny it," he said unable to contain himself. He burst out laughing. Which, of course, got us all laughing.

"I thought we were talking about dieting," I said.

"We are," Adam said. "I just wanted to point out that you really are willing to try anything. Or at least, you were." I nodded and smiled.

"Uh huh."

"At least you can say you started your own diet plan," Adam said regaining his composure. "How many people can say that?"

"You started your own diet plan," Nate said

"Sort of," I said nodding. Then I thought about it. "Well... Not exactly. Like Adam said, I've tried every diet I could ever get my hands on, and most of them have a few things that make sense. My biggest challenge was trying to figure out how to manage a diet. How to manage me, on a diet.

"And, as you know, I'm pretty good at teaching people how to become better managers. Which is what I do for a living; train managers." Adam and Nate nodded. They both know what I do for a living.

"Eventually, I figured out, what I needed to do was to take all the things that I've learned, from all of the diets I tried – plus all of the other things that worked for me – and then manage myself, and my diet, just like I would manage an employee.

"With an employee, I would set up clear goals and expectations.

I would write a job routine so that they knew where they are supposed to be, and when they are supposed to be there. I would make sure that they had all the time, tools and training they needed to get their jobs done and then I would be constantly checking in with them to see their progress and, most importantly, to see if there was any way that I could make it easier for them."

"Serve your staff," Adam said, repeating my daily mantra.

"Exactly," I said. "Except now I'm serving myself. Putting myself first."

"So, you don't follow any diet," Nate said, "or you do; I'm confused." I shook my head.

"No, no. I didn't mean to say that I don't follow a diet plan. I do. I use Weight Watchers. But I also took everything I've learned from all the other diets I've tried, all the "do's and don'ts" and basically wrote myself a job routine. I'm just managing myself better."

"I hate Weight Watchers," Adam said shaking his head in disgust.

"How do you hate Weight Watchers," I said. "You've never even tried it."

"I know," Adam said. "It's the whole point system and tracking, and having to convert everything into a number. I mean, why make it more difficult than it already is."

"Ha," I said, but I knew what he meant. When you're struggling with your weight, I mean, really struggling, (more than 100lbs overweight) everything is difficult. Putting on your shoes, getting in and out of your car, avoiding all the stares and rude comments from other people... not eating junk food, going to the bathroom... everything. It's tough.

Then Weight Watchers comes along and says, "Hey, we can help you lose weight, you just need to learn this whole new language first." And, speaking as a former fat guy, I barely had the energy to get my own work done. The thought of having to learn a new language so that I could try another diet I'm probably not going to be very good at, was... well... I understood what he meant.

"Two things," I said. "First, with the new Weight Watchers plan, I use the app on my phone; there really isn't much you have to learn. Second you don't have to do Weight Watchers," I said. "You should. But you don't have too." Adam smiled and nodded as if he won the argument. He didn't.

"Either way," I said waving off his smile. "If you really want to be successful in losing weight, you have to do two things, regardless of what diet you are going to follow.

"First, pick a diet that is as close to (a) your current eating habits as possible, and (b) your current surroundings. Meaning, I was never successful following Atkins because I grew up eating basically everything, (breads, vegetables, fruits and meat) and cutting three of the four food groups out of my diet was beyond difficult, it was painful. And (b) I also don't live and work in a meat packing plant where I am constantly surrounded by lean meats all day. I work out here," I say gesturing to my surroundings. "And out here I'm surrounded by everything; carbs, fats, proteins, fruits, vegetables, bags of chips, ice cream, pizza...

"And, in my opinion, it is far easier to manage these things, than it is to avoid them." They both nodded in agreement.

"Second."

"That was two," Adam said holding up two fingers.

"No, it wasn't. That one just had two parts."

"Okay," he said. But I knew I was losing him.

"The second thing, and probably the most important thing, Adam; you are going to have to start keeping track of what you eat every day. It doesn't matter if you count carbs, or calories or points; to be successful you need to pay attention and keep track of everything."

"You're probably right," Adam said taking in some air and shuffling around some papers.

"Adam's right," Nate said. "You should write another book." I smiled and nodded.

"Maybe I should."

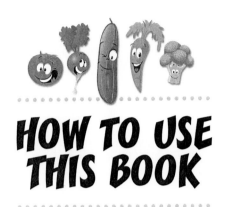

HOW TO USE
THIS BOOK

Before we get too far into this book, I should tell you how to read it, what to expect and why you shouldn't skip ahead. This book is broken up into four parts: Waking Up Fat, Adventures in Dietland, 50 Rules Every One Needs to Know – To Win at the Game of Dieting, & Losing Weight is Not About Losing Weight.

Waking Up Fat: The book begins with a story of credibility. To finally quit smoking (after years and years and years of trying to quit on my own), I took a smoking cessation class. We met once a week, for six weeks and learned how to manage our lives after cigarettes.

Five weeks into the class, someone from the group asked our instructor how long he had smoked before quitting.

"I've never smoked," he said. "I chewed tobacco." There was an audible sigh from the group. He had just lost all credibility and half the class. I'll be honest, I too almost reconsidered. I too, almost didn't try to quit smoking because suddenly, everything that he had taught us, even though it made sense and seemed possible five seconds before, somehow came into question. I remember wanting to call him out on it. To cry foul. I wanted to point out that "chewing tobacco" was not even close to being the same thing as smoking cigarettes. But I didn't. I was already committed to quitting and convinced I could do it. Thank God.

You don't have to worry about this with me. I was really...well... I want to say "heavy" as if that explains it. It doesn't. I was obese. <deep breath> It's still hard to use that word. Obese.

I have tons of pictures on my website www.adventuresindietland. com, to prove it. To show you what I looked like at 350+lbs.... in all my glory. None of the pictures (I assure you) are photo shopped.

I start the book with the story of how I woke up fat, because I want you to know what happened; how it happened; how I got there, and, most importantly, how I was finally able to retake control of my life and lose the weight. The reason for this, of course, is not to brag, but to prove to you that if I can do it, you can do it.

Why listen to me? Why read my books and watch my videos and attend my seminars? Because of credibility. I have been where you are and I know how you feel. It sucks... You hate it... I hated it... This book can help. I can help. Trust me.

Adventures in Dietland: I've tried nearly every diet that I've ever heard about. At least the ones that seemed like they would work. Ones that had actual plans. Everything from Weight Watchers to Jenny Craig to the Paleo Diet and Eating Right for your Blood Type and Herbalife, and on and on and on.

Through this experience, I have learned what works for me and, most importantly, what (and why) most diets didn't. Adventures in Dietland is really more of a synopsis of the good, the bad and the ugly. For instance, the Atkins Diet makes a lot of sense and it works for a lot of people. It didn't work for me because the diet was way too far out of my normal eating habits, and, at 350lbs, I was addicted to sugar.

Of course, I didn't know that I was addicted to sugar when I started stuffing my face with pounds and pounds of chicken and steak and bacon... However, it didn't matter how much protein (or fat) I consumed, I constantly craved bread, and cookies, and pasta and pizza and donuts and bags of potato chips and ice cream and... you get the point. I craved sugar.

Following the Atkins Diet today, after losing more than 150lbs and no longer having an addiction to sugar, is easy peasy. In fact, my current diet closely resembles the Adkins Diet, eating mostly lean proteins and vegetables. But at 350lbs… there was no way I could do it. Oh sure, I would hold out for a couple of weeks, eating just meat and cheese and mayonnaise, but once the Induction phase was over, I would go hog wild and eat every piece of bread in site. In the end, I always ended up gaining more weight than I lost, every time I tried.

Then there is the Grapefruit diet, which seems completely ridiculous – I mean, how can eating grapefruit make you lose weight… right? However, the truth is eating grapefruit (especially when paired with a lean protein) does suppress my appetite. I know… It's crazy, but it works.

50 Rules Every One Needs to Know – To Win at the Game of Dieting: These rules are the crème de le crème. The cream of the cream. The best of the best. The nuts and bolts to how I lost (and have kept off for years), more than 150 lbs. These Rules – some are food related, some are attitude adjusters, some are more bricks and mortar in structure – are the rules I used to manage myself. Manage my diet, my life, my attitude, my space, my cupboards, my decision and eventually, my weight.

Start with the First Ten: Read and follow the first ten Rules. The other 40 Rules can be read and applied in any order. Though I suggest you read through them all the first time, and then continue to browse through, read, digest, share and use all the other Rules that make the most sense to you; I do understand not all Rules are going to apply to everyone.

For instance, "Peeing in the woods," may not be a useful Rule for you to follow if you don't have a long commute to work, and or if you don't find yourself having to stop somewhere to pee on a daily basis. The same can be said about "Quitting the Gym." You may not belong to a gym.

Each Rule, however, stands on their own. It doesn't matter if you can incorporate just one Rule, or all 50 into your life. Begin with the first ten, set yourself up to win and you will see the benefits.

Losing Weight is Not About Losing Weight: In the end, if you are serious about losing weight, then you will have to come to grips with the idea that the same person that allowed you to overeat and put yourself (and your health) last, cannot be the same person who turns your life around. The person who sets you straight, holds you accountable, and kicks your ass every time you get off track. That person still has to be you, of course... but a different you. You will have to change. Or at least, I did.

This book is intended to be eye opening, poignant, and funny. Most of all, I hope this book gives you with all the Rules and knowledge you need to win at the game of dieting. I hope, after reading this book, you are able to (once and for all) throw the game board, the dice, and all the stupid little game pieces in the trash and never have to play again. It's going to take some work, but it's worth it... You are worth it.

CHAPTER ONE

Waking Up Fat

It took a few minutes for me to realize what I was looking at. I had been slowly coming in and out of consciousness for longer than I could comprehend, when I finally decided to open my eyes to see what was preventing me from moving. It was the toilet. I was laying on my left side, with my head firmly stuck between it and the bathtub behind me. My head was pounding, my neck hurt and, to my dismay, my mouth was open.

I struggled, rolling to my right, trying to get up but my hand slipped on what would turn out to be vomit, and I fell back down, twisting my neck even more. I reached up and grabbed the edge of the toilet bowl and tried to figure out where my left arm was. It was under me, asleep and of no use. I took a deep breath and with all of my strength, rolled, lifted, squirmed and twisted myself up to a sitting position. I grabbed my left arm and began to message it back to life as I attempted to shake the cob webs out of my head. I looked around the bathroom. It was empty except for a few towels that were on the floor, soaking up various puddles. The door was open, sun light was coming in from the window in the next room and I was naked.

I think about that morning often. About the way I felt. The shame, the embarrassment, the guilt, the anger... the thoughts of suicide... and all of the events that led up to it. I think about the Booze Cruise, and the Jack Daniels and of always being the life of the party. I think about the security guard that found me rolling on the floor in the public bathroom, unable to get up, but thinking it was hilarious and no big deal.

. . . .

"Just give me a hand up," I said as if this was normal. He did, but told me he had to bring me back to my room; that I had had enough to drink and he needed to get me a nurse.

"I'm cool. I'm cool," I said getting up. "I don't need a nurse." Then I saw myself in the mirror. Blood was running down my face. I reached up to find its source but couldn't.

"You must have taken quite a fall," he said grabbing my waist and putting my arm around his shoulder. I laughed and tried to shrug him off.

"Sir," he said. "Let me help you." I did; until we went outside and I saw all of the people that I was partying with. They were still in the hot tub or at the bar in the pool. A game of pool volleyball was still going on. A few of them noticed us and I immediately got embarrassed. I pulled away from the security guard.

"I'm okay," I said. "I'm going to go with you. Just let me walk on my own." He studied me for a minute and asked me if I was sure. I said I was.

When people ask me about hitting the proverbial "Rock Bottom" I am always cute with my answer. "I didn't just hit rock bottom," I say. "I hit rock bottom and then I fell down the stairs." I say it as if I am joking, but I'm not.

The truth is, I only made it a few feet on my own. Then I fell down a set of concrete steps that led into the pool. The security guard, in full uniform, had to come in and get me. As he pulled me out of the pool and walked me back to my room, past everyone that I had been hanging out with for the last 3 days, I stared at the ground, wishing I was someone else, somewhere else. In that moment, I truly hated myself.

It was 8pm on Wednesday, April 24, 2013 at the beautiful, all-inclusive Breezes Resort in Nassau Bahamas. I was there celebrating my 42nd birthday. I weighed more than 350lbs and if you couldn't tell from this introduction, I had a pretty bad drinking problem; I was obesely overweight and I was miserable.

This was not the first time I woke up fat, alone, hung over, miserable, hating myself, my life, and literally everything in between. The truth is, I have woken up fat many times.

There was this one time when I was flying to State College Pennsylvania for a company meeting when I was singled out by the flight attendant. 'We need to ask a couple of people to take a different flight because the plane is too heavy,' she said. I remember her standing in front of me, making the announcement more to me, than anyone else. I looked at her and was not really getting what she was saying, but thinking, 'I'm not taking another flight.' But before I could respond someone from behind me said, "If he gets off, then that will be enough right." The flight attendant pursed her lips together and nodded, then looked back at me.

"Well?" She said. I looked at her, and started to turn back toward the person behind me when it dawned on me. She singled me out because "I" was too heavy for the plane. I nodded.

"Well," I agreed, and got off the plane.

Flying always sucked for me. No one ever wanted to sit beside me and I would spend the entire flight sucking my stomach in and trying my hardest not to take up more space than I was supposed to; which was always easier said than done, and seat belts... Ugh... don't get me started on seatbelts.

I had a strategy for putting on my seat belt. I would literally lift my stomach up and tuck the seat belt in the fold, where my belt was hiding, and then suck in as much as I could while fumbling with the clasp. It worked 99% of the time. Except for this one time when I was flying to Chicago. I was going through the normal routine of lifting my stomach, tucking in the seat belt and fumbling for the clasp, when the flight attendant saw me and in the most sarcastic tone, and loudest, booming voice, said, "You know that is not going to work. I am going to have to get you a seat belt extender." I could feel my face instantly start to burn with embarrassment and I wanted to die, right there on the spot.

I was in a business meeting once, in a large conference room with about 12 other people. We were all sitting around in neatly pressed suites, highly polished shoes and discussing financial models when I leaned back in my chair and it broke, sending me ass over backwards and onto the floor. It happened in slow motion, of course. I leaned back, the chair buckled and then there was a loud snapping sound and everyone looked up from the table just in time to watch me tumble over backwards. By the time I got up everyone had turned away and tried their best not to laugh out loud. Someone suggested that we take a five-minute break so that I could find another chair and everyone ran out of the room quickly, unable to stifle their laughter any longer. I spent the rest of the meeting thinking about ways that I could kill myself without it hurting too much.

My doctor sent me to see a specialist once, and when I got there it turned out that the "Specialist" was a Type II Diabetes specialist. Perplexed I said, "But I don't have Type II diabetes." She checked my chart, saw that I was right and then slowly looked me over from head to toe.

"You will soon enough," she said and told me to sit down. I did.

There was this other time that I drove by a car accident. It wasn't too big of an accident, but it had just happened and the driver's side door was caved in. A couple of guys, who were driving by at the same time, ran over and helped pull the guy out of his driver side window.

I remember watching and thinking that there was no way that anyone could have pulled me out of my own car window. That if I got in an accident, they would have to use the Jaws of Life to cut me out of my car. That was a scary realization. I drove a small car and even with my seat pushed all the way back, the steering wheel was still only a couple of inches away from my belly.

From that point on I couldn't shake the feeling that if I got into an accident, even a small one, I would be trapped. I was too fat to get out of my own car. I didn't even get out of my car like a normal person. I had to put my hand on the ground and sort of roll out of my car.

There was this other time when I was picking up an order of Chinese food, and the lady behind the counter asked if I wanted plates, forks and napkins with my order. I said yes and she started counting out six plates, and six forks...

"No, no," I said stopping her. "I just need one of each."

"One of each," she repeated, in disbelief. She looked at the paper bag that was full to the top of all the greats, Pork Fried Rice, Crab Rangoon, Boneless Spareribs, General Tso Chicken, a couple of Spring Rolls, and of course my favorite, Chicken Fingers, and then she looked back at me. She gave me the most disgusted look. "What?" I thought. It's just lunch.

I didn't even put it together until after I got home and saw that she had given me six fortune cookies. I was eating for six! My dumb ass.

I have hundreds of stories like this. Hundreds of times when I realized how fat I was. Which is an interesting statement because despite weighing more than 350lbs (at only 6' tall), and having a 20-inch neck and a 48-inch waste, I didn't always realize I was heavy. I avoided mirrors for the most part, and was really, really good at making up excuses and lying to myself.

. . . .

So why now you ask. Why this day? What was so different on this day than any other? How did I go from being both completely oblivious and a big fat liar to just being fat on the morning of April 25, 2013? How was I finally able to, not just declare that I've had enough, but to actually do something about it?

I have asked myself this question a million times and have narrowed the answer down to a mixture of four things: Timing, a Clear View, a Witness and good old fashioned Fear.

CHAPTER TWO

Timing is Everything

I like to say that everything snuck up on me. The 150 extra pounds I was carrying around, the drinking problem, my forties. The truth, however, as much as I tried to keep my head in the sand and lie, I knew what was happening. I knew I was out of control. That I was going to have to get my act together, I knew that my forties were coming, that my ass was growing, that my drinking was getting more and more out of control, and if I was ever going to be the person I had always dreamed of being, I would have to change. The question was, when. When was I going to get my act together? When was I going to stop eating and drinking like it didn't matter. Like I didn't matter. When was I going to start doing all the things that I had so desperately wanted to do and stop doing all the things that I didn't.

On June 17th, 2007 I wrote the number 1,394 on a white board I had hanging in my office. It was how many days I had until my 40th birthday. I remember figuring the number out. Counting the rest of the days left in June, then the rest of the year, adding three years to that number and then the remaining 102 days until my birthday in 2011.

At the time I thought it was going to be in the thousands, not just barely over one thousand. The number seemed so small. Like my 40's were right around the corner. It was as if my 30's were already over. I remember standing there staring at it and then calculating it again to make sure I was right. I was.

The number made me nervous. I had so many things that I wanted to do before I turned 40. So many things that I needed to do. I wrote down the following "Things to do by the time I'm 40," list.

- Become a "real" writer / author – publish a book, or ten
- Have millions of dollars in the bank
- Earn a Master's Degree
- Run the Vermont City Marathon
- Quit my job – Start my own company

- Start teaching / training people how to become managers
- Lose weight – Get healthy
- Quit drinking
- Be happy
- Inspire others

Fast forward 2,137 days, on the morning of April 25, 2013, more than 2 years after my 40th birthday and I woke up being further away from those goals than I could have ever imagined. Instead of making the best of those 1,394 days, I continued to bury my head in the sand. I continued to over eat, to over drink, to dream without action and I didn't complete a single goal on my list.

. . . .

The room we were staying in was on the 6th floor and had a small balcony that faced the courtyard of the resort. The pool, with the swim up bar and volley ball net, was in the center. Two huge hot tubs were beyond that, overlooking the ocean and the public bathroom, a small concrete building, was even further back, off to the left. In the distance the clear blue green ocean slowly ebbed and flowed.

I know this is going to sound crazy but I have fallen from a couple buildings in my life; once when I was a kid playing with my brother at an abandoned factory, and another while working in construction. Ever since that second one, I have had a tough time with heights and generally avoided things like balconies.

I slowly walked to the door of the balcony and looked out at everything, though I can't say that I was really seeing anything. I just kept replaying the night before, the week before, the months and months and years before... all the drinking and eating and careless behavior. All the missed opportunities... all the time wasted and all the dreams... so many dreams. Dreams of being an author, a motivational speaker, of being healthier and happier; of not being so fat and miserable.

Instead I was standing on a balcony, in the middle of paradise, wishing I had the nerve to jump. To take just two steps out the door and hurdle myself over the railing. But I couldn't bring myself to do it. I knew what falling felt like and it made me sick to my stomach. Besides, hitting the ground really hurts and I was already in enough pain.

CHAPTER THREE

Can I Get a Witness?

A couple of months before the trip to the Bahamas I had been on a four or five, (maybe even six) week bender. That is, I drank every single night, whether I was out with friends, at home with my wife, or alone in a hotel room, I drank.

I didn't realize it at first, that I had been drinking every day, for weeks, until the night of the trade show. I worked in sales for a large management company and I attended a lot of trade shows where, letting your hair down and getting liquored up is more than just expected; it's the normal course of business.

The night before the trade show, having too much work to catch up on to go out, Jack (Daniels) and I stayed in the hotel room and half worked, half channel surfed and stayed up way too late, drinking way too much. I slept through the first two morning sessions, missed a conference call with my boss and barely made it down in time for the trade show start, at 11am.

"You look terrible," a friend said when she saw me. "Who did you go out with last night?" I smiled and tried to quickly pull out a couple of names of people that I could have gone out with but no one came to mind.

"What are you asking me," I said instead of answering her. I didn't want to admit that I spent the night drinking alone. She laughed and said everyone was meeting at the bar at 2:30, after the trade show, and that I owed her a drink for some reason.

"Okay," I agreed but the thought of going to the bar, of drinking more alcohol, of retelling the same old stories, and of always being the life of the party, made my stomach turn. 'There is no way I am going to the bar,' I thought. I just wanted to go home.

I remember standing at my booth and trying to figure out the last time that I hadn't had a drink. Had it really been weeks? More than a month? The realization was more than depressing, it was embarrassing. I never wanted to be this person.

I promised myself I was not going to the bar, was not going to drink that night; and in fact, if I had anything to say about it, I wasn't going to drink anymore. Ever. But by the time the trade show ended I had eaten, drank a bunch of water, taken aspirin and was feeling better. Besides, all of my current clients, future clients, and fellow vendors were going to the bar and so it felt more like a work event than just a trip to the bar, and if it was work event, then I was obligated. So I went.

The next day, Friday, I got home around 6pm and found my wife on the back deck drinking a beer, smoking a cigarette and on the phone with a girlfriend. "I bought you some more Jack," she said. "It's in the bag on the counter, but I think you still have some in the cupboard." She kissed me on the cheek. I took a deep breath and sat down. The last thing I wanted was more Jack Daniels.

When she got off the phone she sat down beside me and we talked about our week. I'm a story teller at heart and I often embellish here and there, adding just enough humor to make my days seem a lot funnier than they actually are. On this day, however, I told the truth. I told her about my drinking, even when I was alone in a hotel room, and about the night before. Despite how I was feeling when I woke up, I went to the bar anyway; and about the dinner plans I made with clients for 6:30pm and how I didn't make it past 5:30 before the bartender shut me off.

"You should have seen me," I told her. "I was a mess. I am still a mess. I didn't even make it to the dinner."

She assured me it probably wasn't as bad as I thought it was.

That everyone drinks at these things and that no one would judge me, and even if they did; F' them, she said and then she went inside and made me a drink.

"I'm serious," I said when she came out with it. "I've got to stop drinking."

"Then don't drink it," she said setting it down beside me and opening herself another beer.

If only she'd been there, I thought. If only she had seen me. Had witnessed how much I drank, and not just last night, but every night and how stupid I look and how foolish I behave. Then she would understand. She would see that I was out of control, that I needed help. She would help.

By the end of that weekend I had formulated a plan. I was going to get my life back on track. I was going to rejoin Weight Watchers; I was going to start walking until I could run, and then I was going to start running; I was going to go back to school, signing back up for my Master's Degree... again (I had started and dropped out twice already) and I was going to quit drinking. On Sunday night, while eating Chinese take-out, I told her about my plans.

She took it all in stride, nonchalantly nodding her head between bites of Sweet and Sour Chicken. "And when are you going to do all of this," she said. I had made such declarations before and she wasn't all that convinced.

"Weight Watchers and walking," I said. "Tomorrow. School... I have to look into, and drinking... April 19th."

She laughed at that. Twelve years earlier, April 19, 2001 I quit smoking cigarettes. I had just turned 30 years old (on the 12th), and I was smoking more than two packs a day at the time. I had been smoking since I was 14 or 15 years old, and my dad had just been diagnosed with emphysema the year prior.

Ever since, April 19th has been a very important day to me. It was the first day that I was able to take control of my life. To beat an addiction that I had previously thought was impossible to beat, and it seemed fitting to use that day as the day I would do it again, this time with drinking. It was March 22nd.

My wife continued eating and nodding, knowing the significance of that day and then she took out her phone and looked at her calendar.

"You know that is the weekend that we are going to the Bahamas, for your birthday," she said. I confessed that I didn't remember. That I hadn't even thought about it. I remember her saying how ridiculous it was that I wanted to try to quit drinking during the week I was going to be at an all-inclusive (i.e. free Jack Daniels) resort in the Bahamas. "It's like trying to start a diet on the morning of Thanksgiving," she said. She was always a funny girl and to my regret, I agreed.

. . . .

It was almost 1pm by the time I had stopped crying, dry heaving and feeling suicidal long enough to shower and make my way down stairs to find some aspirin, food and my wife. She was out by the pool sunbathing.

Before I could say anything to her, a couple of guys that I had met the day before (on the Booze Cruise) saw me and came over. They were surprised to see me, saying that they heard I had been arrested for throwing a cop in the pool.

"He didn't throw a cop in the pool," my wife said looking up and shielding her eyes with her hand. "The cop had to jump in the pool to rescue him."

"Wow," they said. "Holy shit. You were pretty drunk."

I didn't know what to say to that, so I didn't say anything. I tried to smile and nod my head, but even the slightest movement was making me noxious.

"You know what you need," one of them said. "You need a little hair of the dog." I shook my head slowly.

"No chance," I said softly.

"He's probably right," my wife said getting up. "A drink will make you feel better." I remember looking at her and not believing what I was hearing.

"I will never drink again," I said shaking my head. "Never, ever, ever..."

"Don't say that," she said. "Maybe just don't drink so much today." Then she gathered up her stuff and started walking toward the buffet. "Let's go get lunch," she said. I remember standing there, in the blazing sun, my head pounding, my stomach all twisted up in knots, both of my knees were scraped raw, my face, right shoulder and hands were all cut up and I wished, more than anything, that I had the energy to yell.

"Didn't you see me last night!" I wanted to scream. "Can't you see me now! I am cut up from head to toe. I had to be rescued and escorted back to the hotel room from a security guard. They had to have a nurse come and check on me every couple of hours to make sure I was still alive. I woke up French kissing the base of a toilet and if that wasn't bad enough I just spent the last 60 minutes trying to get the nerve to throw myself from the God damned balcony!" But I didn't.

She got to the door of the restaurant before she realized I wasn't following her. She turned back toward me looking exasperated. "Are you coming," she said impatiently.

I took in some air, wanted to shake my head no, but then followed her anyway.

CHAPTER FOUR

A Clear View

The Resort gave you two options if you wanted to sit outside and drink by the pool. You could be in the pool, sitting at the bar on concrete bar stools or you could be on the deck, sitting in wooden high back stools. Like most people, I started on the deck and eventually made my way into the pool – the whole-time meeting and talking to everyone. I was in rare form.

It didn't matter who you were or what you were doing, I would smile, drink, and introduce myself. I work in sales, and have always considered my job, and hence myself, as a professional visitor... and I love to visit.

"You know you don't have to be in everyone's conversation," a guy at the bar said. I could feel the smile slowly leave my face as I looked up. He was shirtless, sunglasses on his head, arms full of tattoos. He stared at me, blank faced at first and then his expression changed. He closed his eyes, raised his hands and began pretending that he was talking to everyone on his left, and then everyone on his right. He shook his head back and forth, pretending he was talking to everyone around him, mocking me.

I remember sitting there, with a dumb look on my face, staring at him; trying to comprehend what he was talking about and what he was doing. But then I got it. I looked back at the three ladies to my left, the ones who were just a minute ago, talking among themselves, until I tried to interject myself into their conversation and this guy, Tattoo, called me on it. They had all found their phones and kept their heads down, avoiding the confrontation. I felt like a big, fat, stupid, ass. I grabbed my drink and made my way into the pool. It was Tuesday, April 23, 2013; two days before I would wake up, fat.

. . . .

This wasn't the first time I had been called out for trying to be in everyone's conversation. A friend of mine called me out at a bar once, years before and the memory of it still stung.

"You're just looking pathetic," he said under his breath so only I could hear. "Like you're trying too hard." I remember my face feeling hot and my ears burning with embarrassment. I looked away and ordered another Jack Daniels.

"On the rocks," I said, no longer needing the soda chaser. I knew how I looked. Fat, dumb, ugly, drunk, slow, pathetic, not nearly as smart as I thought I was, sloppy, loud, with bad taste, a shit pallet, narcissistic, self-important, unaware, unkempt, awkward and a fucking know-it-all.

I knew all of it. And to be honest, I thought I did a good job at hiding it all too. Locking it away, so that no one else had to look at it. The problem, of course, is the only person I was fooling was me.

. . . .

It didn't take too long, an hour maybe, but eventually the pool and the bar filled up with vacationers from all over the world; everyone was eager to have a good time. I forgot tattoo, the three ladies at the bar, and how obnoxious I looked to everyone around me. I resumed talking too much, laughing too loud, drinking more than I should be, and getting into everyone's conversation.

Fast forward 24 hours and I am being escorted into the hotel, through a piano bar and past that same group of women. They are at the piano, drinks in hand, singing at the top of their lungs, "My Life," by Billy Joel. They turn, along with everyone else in the bar, when we walk in. I'm wearing only a pair of shorts, no shirt. The security guard and I are soaking wet and I am bleeding from head to toe. I remember trying my hardest to not look up. Not to see them seeing me, but I can't help it. I'm hoping they don't look, but they do. They stand, half turned, looking at me. Their mouths open in disbelief. One of them laughing and pointing at me. "OMG! Do you remember that guy," she said?

It's was one of the most humiliating and disturbing times in my life. I can still see their faces. Their expressions. It was as if they were mirrors and looking at them, looking at me, gave me a clear view of who I really was. I could no longer avoid the truth. Could no longer bury my head in the sand and pretend that I wasn't as fat as I was. Wasn't as loud and obnoxious as I was. Wasn't as drunk and desperate as I was. Wasn't as pathetic as I was... I needed to change.

. . . .

Everything hurt the next morning. The bottoms of my feet, from playing too much pool volleyball, my knees, shoulder and the palms on both hands from falling in the bathroom and then in the pool. My head, my stomach, even my left ear, which I had somehow scraped against some concrete. The thing that hurt the most, however was my pride. My ego. It was as if my self-identity had been dragged across a large piece of 60 grit sandpaper. It was left open and raw.

But it wasn't until I walked back downstairs; until I saw those two guys. Until I saw how they saw me. Small, wounded, pathetic, weak, fat, drunk, hopeless... It was like pouring salt on my wounds. That is when I remembered Tattoo and the women from the pool side bar (and later, the piano bar), and my friend trying to give me a head's up without embarrassing me.

How many more times did I have to see myself, as I really am. As others saw me, before I had had enough? How many more times was I going to act like an asshole before I decided that I no longer wanted to be an asshole? When was I going to start deciding who I wanted to be? Deciding what kind of person, I wanted to be; instead of just acting like it doesn't matter... like I don't matter.

CHAPTER FIVE

Scared Shitless

I can still recall the nauseous feeling. The sickness that burned in my stomach and continuously made me wretch, even though there was nothing left to expel. The headache that seemed to start from somewhere above me and radiate like pulsing waves through my head. Top to bottom. Top to bottom. The tingling feeling in my fingers and toes and the spinning. The room would not stop spinning. I remember trying to open my eyes and focus on something, anything. Just trying to get the room to stop spinning, but the light. The light was so bright, that I couldn't do it. I couldn't open my eyes wide enough to focus on anything. I held on and prayed, and dry heaved, and hoped and promised... If I made it out of this – I thought. If I made it through the night; if I lived to see another day, I would give up drinking, I would stop eating like an asshole, I would take control of my life... I promise.

The next morning, still reeling from the night before, I couldn't shake the dreadful feeling that I was going to die being the same person, in the same place, doing the same things, with all my dreams and aspirations - left unfulfilled. As if dying wasn't bad enough, the thought of dying because I couldn't take control of my own actions, made it ten times worse.

When I was 17 I started working for a masonry company as a laborer. I did it for eight years and I hated it. At one point the Foreman asked me if I wanted to learn how to become a Mason. I could join the union and carve out a pretty good life for myself, he told me. I wasn't so sure. I worked with a guy named Charlie. He was 40 years old, had been a mason for 20 years and took pain medication three times a day due to the heavy receptiveness of picking up bricks and mortar eight hours a day, five days a week.

Charlie was the type of guy who would stop working at 3:00pm every day. He would spend the next 30 minutes cleaning his tools, and making his way to the shop trailer we had on site. At 3:30pm he would head to the closest convenience store and grab a six-pack of beer. Although he lived only 30 or 40 minutes away from the site, he would drink the entire six-pack before stopping at another convenience store, this one right around the corner from his house, and grab another.

Once home he would yell at the neighbor kids for playing on his lawn. Maybe he would play a quick game of fetch with his dog. Then he'd eat dinner in front of the television and eventually pass out on the couch – only to wake up the next day and do it all over again.

More than the fear of dying, or of getting type II diabetes, (which is very common in my family) or of falling in the bathtub (I read somewhere that a person who is more than 100lbs overweight is more likely to die from falling in the tub, than a person who isn't overweight). Like I needed that information in my life.

More than all of that, I was scared shitless of turning out to be just like Charlie. Just like everyone else I had known. Everyone who believed that they didn't have any choices. That they weren't smart enough or strong enough; that it didn't matter... that they didn't matter.

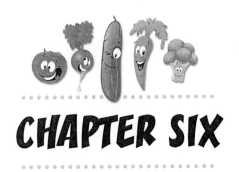

CHAPTER SIX

Adventures in Dietland: Let the Games Begin

"Ralph. We need to talk about Jenny." I knew this conversation was coming. I had seen the looks; the eye rolls, the exasperation, her head shaking back and forth every time Jenny showed up. I've heard the muttering under her breath, and knew she thought I was being ridiculous. Heck, I knew that I was being ridiculous. But I didn't want to talk about Jenny. Not today. I had just called for a delivery and a couple of pizzas, two dozen boneless wings, and some of their new cinnamon sticks, were on their way to my front door at that very moment. I looked up at her and smiled sheepishly.

"I know," I said trying to end the conversation before it started.

"No," she said. "You don't. The mice have gotten into them and, from what I can tell, Jenny isn't helping them lose weight either." We both started laughing. "I'm serious." She said. "We're going to have to get bigger mouse traps." She sat down on the couch across from me, but she didn't sit back. She sat with her arms on her knees. It was her, "we need to talk" position. I was reclining in the lazy boy, channel surfing. I sat up, but didn't want to.

"I'm going to start eating them." She rolled her eyes. "I am," I said. She took a deep breath. It was no longer funny. She was serious. "I'm just not ready to stop."

"Yeah... well, you have too." We looked at each other for a full minute. Neither of us blinking. Then she sat back. "How much longer," she said. "I mean, honestly. How much more money are we going to spend before you realize it isn't going to work?" She paused. "When was the last time you ate any of that stuff anyway? Honestly?" I thought about it, but couldn't remember and looked away.

This wasn't the first time that I had signed up to have meals delivered to my house, so that I could "Grab and Go" without any thought or effort. Jenny was just the last straw.

· · · · · · · · · · · · ·

Around the time, I turned 14 or 15, we got a microwave. It was this huge clunky box that sounded like a vacuum cleaner was stuck inside a closet. My mom had just started working evenings at a food supply warehouse, and the combination of these two things (the microwave and my mom's work), would have a profound effect on me.

One year earlier, my sister (a year older than me) was in the kitchen with our mom nearly every day, learning how to cook, clean, scrub, measure, problem solve, check meat temperatures, etc. Not me. There wasn't room for more than two people in our tiny kitchen and I would have to wait my turn – a turn that never came. Instead we got a microwave, and mom started working nights.

This is in 1985 – 1986, and the microwave oven revolution was exploding. So much so that the food supply warehouse that my mother worked at began carrying all the latest "Microwavable Food." There were Hot Pockets, and French Bread Pizza, and Microwaveable TV Dinners, and Pizza Bites, and Pot Pies, and Popcorn... Tons and tons of Popcorn.

My mom, working nights and no longer having the time to cook, began bringing this stuff home by the bag full. For the next few years our freezer would be chocked full of bright red and yellow boxes, and I ate all of it. Ramen noodles and microwavable cheeseburgers, and "Micro Magic" French fries and cheese covered casseroles and Bagel Bites.

Suddenly, as if overnight, we turned into a "grab and go" family.

I went from complaining, "Mom, I'm hungry," and her saying back, "You're going to have to wait until dinner," to no longer having to ask, or wait. If I was hungry, I went to the freezer, pulled out whatever looked good, popped it into the microwave, and that was it. Sometimes it was a snack, like Bagel Bites, and sometimes it was full Hungry Man meal. I had no control. I ate when I wanted, as much as I wanted.

In retrospect, it is easy to see how or why I gained so much weight. I had lost all patience with hunger as a teenager. Couple that with my inability to cook anything, and then add on top of that all the food that is readily available for order, takeout or as a diet plan, and poof... Fat City.

This is the crux of the problem with diet plans that send me food, or meal replacement shakes, it only exacerbated my problem. It didn't help me gain more patience with hunger. It didn't teach me how to put meals together, or how to cook; and worse, they told me that I didn't have to worry about counting calories, or tracking points, or paying attention to carbs.

Instead they said, "We know you're busy. We know you don't have time to plan every meal and cook. You're tired... You've worked all day. Let us do it for you."

You know who else has that same sales pitch? McDonald's, Burger King, Wendy's, KFC, your local Chinese takeout, Domino's Pizza, and the million other fast food restaurants that are promising you delicious food, fast.

"We know you're busy," They say, commiserating with you. "We know you don't have the time, or the energy. We know that you've worked all day... Don't worry. We'll even feed the kids and give them a toy – you won't even have to get out of the car."

Eventually, I put all this together and concluded that if I was serious about changing my life, I needed to learn how to cook. I needed to learn how to plan meals, and pay attention to what I'm eating, and to keep track. I needed to increase my patience with food. I needed to stop listening to every whim my body throws at me (Rule #22), and most importantly, I needed to throw away my microwave (Rule #21).

. . . .

I know I sort of touched on the Atkins diet in the beginning of this book, but let me tell you something... I LOVED being on Atkins. I loved the idea of a diet that had no limits. I loved being able to eat as much steak and chicken and mayonnaise as I wanted.

I read the entire book and understood the science. It made complete sense to me. The problem I had with it, as I've already pointed out, was that it was way too far off from my normal eating routine. I couldn't sustain eating just meat for two weeks, let alone, the idea of eating meat, and only meat, for the rest of my life. And worse, if I did go two weeks (which is what you are supposed to do), I would be compelled to dive head first into a loaf of bread as soon as my two weeks were up. I'd earned it, I thought. Then I'd gain all the weight back. Usually more.

· · · · · · · · · · · ·

This leads me to think about the Paleo Diet, which is a lot like the Atkins Diet in the sense that it tells you to avoid all processed carbs (bread, cakes, cupcakes, pizza, etc.), because early Cave Man didn't have access to such luxuries.

The Paleo Diet, if you don't know, has you eating everything that would have been available to the Cave Man only. Meaning, it is basically a high protein diet, with fruits, vegetables and some nuts. (I bet you've never seen a fat Cave man before, have you? ... Oh, wait, does Captain Caveman count – He's chubby.)

Two things struck me about this diet. First, (apparently) Cave Men didn't have a lot of access to any kind of bird eggs, so if you are going to follow this diet, then you are supposed to eat eggs in moderation. There goes breakfast!

Second, and this really highlights the absurdity in the way I dieted, the Paleo Diet says that you can eat dark chocolate. Dark chocolate! Seriously! The reason for this is because it is believed that early man would have had access to cacao leaves. You couple that little tidbit of information with all the health benefits of dark chocolate and soon, I was eating a large bar of dark chocolate every night. (PS: They only sell large bars of dark chocolate... That's how they get you... It's like buying a pack of 12 hot dog buns, when you only need 10.)

Do you see the absurdity? If you give me an inch, I will take a mile while munching on dark chocolate and pepperoni chips (pepperoni chips... an Atkins staple) every time.

The problem I have with these kind of diets is that they are 99% restrictive on everything you eat, but then there is this tiny loop hole. This little opening that makes the correlation between early man and cacao leaves and poof, I'm going through dark chocolate bars like I'm searching for a Golden Ticket (bonus points if you get that reference).

I didn't even like dark chocolate, but like I said; give me an inch and I will take a mile. I never had any success on the Paleo Diet, except I did start to like dark chocolate – so that's a thing.

. . . .

Today there are a ton of workout video's and programs that are geared toward people who have very little experience in lifting weights, or working out and eating right. In the late 90's the biggest one of these had to be a program called, "Body for Life." The intention behind the program was to get you to become a body builder in 12 short weeks – a habit (they believed) you would continue "For Life."

On this program, you were supposed to eat six times a day, work out (at max intensity) three days a week, while running like you stole something the other three days a week. Then there were Sundays.

Oh, how I loved Sundays. The BFL program was extremely restrictive (just like all the other ones that didn't work for me).

They told you what to eat, what supplements and meal replacement shakes to drink (both of which you would buy from them), when to work out and how. In exchange, they gave you Sundays.

I'd start thinking about Sundays by Tuesday or Wednesday; start planning which fast food joint I wanted to visit by Thursday and by Friday night, I would have an outline drawn up – strategically planning my meals for the entire day. You could eat whatever you wanted, and as much as you wanted, on Sundays. I was in my glory.

Then the 12-week challenge ended and so did my motivation. I lost. I don't mean weight. Though I did lose some weight. A lot really. Something like 45lbs, which at the time, was amazing. I mean I lost the competition. I didn't go from a blubbering fat guy, to a ripped Greek God. All that work, all those early mornings, and lifting heavy stuff and then putting it down, and running so fast I thought I was going to have a heart attack... for nothing. It wasn't enough to win.

See, BFL is a competition. And in this competition, there are no participation medals. You either win, or you don't. For me, that was extremely demotivating. I had no idea that I wouldn't win. I truly worked my ass off. And I didn't get anything for it. I know, I know... I lost 45lbs and got in decent shape... yada, yada, yada... The truth is, because it was sold to me as a competition, a competition that I had a chance of winning, that when I didn't win, nothing else mattered. I got so mad that instead of going to the gym, I went to McDonalds. "F' them," I thought. "F' me!"

Rule #45, sign up for a foot race... one that gives away participation medals. It can be as little as a 5k and as much as a full marathon. Walk until you can run and when you can run (or walk) far enough, enter a foot race and earn yourself a medal. Then hang it on the wall where everyone can see it. It's worth it!

. . . .

I always felt a certain amount of embarrassment with dieting. I hated the idea of telling someone that I was on a diet or talking to someone about it. Not because I was embarrassed that I was trying to get my act together, but because I had a proven record of losing some and then gaining more. Lose some, gain more. It was embarrassing... but Kelly was looking amazing.

"Oh my God, Ralph. It's Weight Watchers," she said when I told her how great she was looking. I had heard of WW, of course, but I didn't quite understand it – the whole counting points thing. So I asked her.

She explained the whole program to me. How everything was converted to a points system. That it was easy once you got the hang of it, and that it worked as long as you kept track of everything you ate. "Tracking is key," she said (Rule #7).

I remember the first time I went to a Weight Watchers meeting. Let me tell you, walking into that place wasn't easy. I felt completely out of place, and didn't think it was for me. Honestly, I thought it was a program for women. I remember sitting in my car; watching people go in. First it was a stream of women. Then a girl. Then two more women and a girl. A grandmother. And then another grandmother, then another. I took a deep breath and got out of the car. Across the parking lot was another guy sitting in a pickup truck. We looked at each other for a moment and then I went in. A few minutes later, he followed.

. . . .

"Ralph, what the hell is this," my friend John said pulling the WW sliding scale Pointsfinder out of my back pocket. We were at a bar waiting for a table. I snatched it back out of his hands, completely embarrassed.

"It's a WW thing," I said. I could feel my ears start to burn. I turned back to the bar and grabbed my drink (Jack Daniels and Diet Coke – 4 points).

"You don't have to do that anymore," he said. "You're skinny now." I smiled at him and drank. It's true, I thought. I have lost a lot of weight. I did feel amazing. I had just broken 300 and weighed around 280lbs. "You're skinny now..."

By the time we got to our table I was feeling lighter and lighter. Or maybe it was the Jack Daniels (two more – 8 points). "You're skinny now."

I remember looking at the menu; at all the gourmet cheeseburgers... they even had Tator Tots (still my favorite). "You're skinny now." The phrase continued like an echo in my mind and I ate like an asshole. I stopped tracking and attending meetings, "I'm skinny now," and I ate whatever I wanted.

A year or so later I would wake up on April 25th, fat... again.

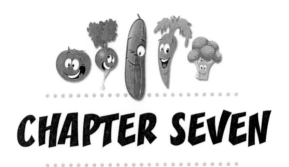

CHAPTER SEVEN

50 Rules Every One Needs to Know

By now, I think you get the point. I've tried a lot of diets and learned a lot of things. Some of the things I've learned were useful, and some not so useful. Every diet has a loop hole. Every diet has a learning curve. Every diet has a different approach to getting you to where you want to be. I'm sure they all work. You just have to find one that works for you.

Personally, my adventure has been long and arduous. Sometimes painful, sometimes frustrating and worst of all, most of the time... ineffective. Until... Well... Until I learned the Rules of dieting.

'Rules,' you say? Oh yes, there are rules. In fact, not knowing the rules – not knowing how to play this game of dieting, is the very reason I have been so terrible at it, and why I never won. Until now.

There are hundreds, perhaps even thousands of rules when it comes to the game of dieting. I have fifty.

"Start peeing in the woods... Burn your fat clothes... Stop supporting the troops... Quit the gym... Get new friends... and every time you think of pushups, do pushups... it doesn't matter if it is one pushup or a hundred... Just do it."

You will not find Rules like these anywhere else, but trust me, following these rules has helped me regain control over my life, my health and my weight.

As stated in the "How to Use this Book" section, begin with the first ten Rules. The other 40 Rules can be read and applied in any order. Though I suggest you read through them all the first time, and then continue to browse through, read, digest, share and use all the other Rules that make the most sense to you; I do understand not all Rules are going to apply to everyone.

For instance, "Peeing in the woods," may not be a useful Rule for you to follow if you don't have a long commute to work, and or if you don't find yourself having to stop somewhere to pee on a daily basis. The same can be said about "Quitting the Gym." You may not belong to a gym.

Each Rule, however, stands on their own. It doesn't matter if you can incorporate just one Rule, or all 50 into your life. Begin with the first ten, set yourself up to win and you will see the benefits.

THE 50 RULES

1. Begin with the End
2. Pick a Start Date
3. Start on Friday
4. Choose a Plan
5. Learn Everything About that Plan
6. Do the Math
7. Track Your Food
8. Get to know Your Doctor
9. Get on the Scale
10. Toughen Up
11. Quit the Gym
12. Do the Dishes
13. Pee in the Woods
14. Burn Your Fat Clothes
15. Waste Your Food
16. Doggy Bags are for Dogs
17. Talk to Yourself
18. Set an Alarm
19. Get New Friends
20. Think About Push Ups
21. Throw Away Your Microwave
22. Stop Listening to Your Body
23. Diet Like it is Your Job
24. Create a Sense of Urgency
25. Stalk Thin People
26. Stop Supporting the Troops
27. Stay Off the Grass
28. Jump, Scream, Curse!
29. Stop Treating every Meal as if it is your Last
30. Put Yourself First
31. Pre-Game
32. Stay away... from Buffets...
33. Use Chop Sticks

1. BEGIN WITH THE END

"What do you want to look like? How do you want to feel? How do you want everyone else to look at you? What kind of a person do you want to be?" These are the questions that I began with. I wrote them down and tried my best to figure out the answers.

"I want be healthy and happy," I wrote. "I don't even care about how much I weigh, as much as I care about how I look. About how I feel.

"I want to be athletic and thin. I want people to take one look at me and know that I take care of myself. That I work out, that I'm fit and athletic. I want to be that forty-something-year-old guy that doesn't look like he's in his forties.

I worked at a radio station once and we had a guest on named

"The Logger." His whole persona was that he was this rugged out-doorsman that talked straight, with an old Vermonter sensibility. He was always polite but never pulled any punches. Oh, and he was as fit as could be, with perfect six-pack abs.

I remember a fan of his showed up at the radio station with homemade cookies. "I don't know if you eat cookies," she said. "I hope you do. I made these special."

I remember watching him with her. A wide grin. A gentleman. He took the plate of cookies even though we all knew he didn't eat cookies.

"I want to be like him," I wrote. "I want to be the type of person that doesn't eat cookies. Or, at least, the type of person who doesn't look like they eat cookies."

"Imagine if someone had to ask you if you ate cookies, because you were in such good shape that you didn't look like you have ever had one in your whole life?" -That's what I wanted.

Beginning with the end is goal setting 101. I didn't just want to lose weight. I wanted to become a different person. I wanted to be the type of person who didn't need alcohol to have a good time. I wanted to be athletic – finding a sport that I liked, could do, and was good at. I wanted to be thin. I wanted to wear stylish clothes and shop at stylish stores.

I ripped the ass in my pants once, on my way to a meeting and had to stop at a store to buy new ones. The only store in town, however, was this hip little place that didn't carry anything over a size 36. I was a size 46. I bought a needle and thread instead and was 20 minutes late to the meeting, while I sat in my car and sewed.

I wanted to have more confidence. I wanted to stand up straighter, to be taken more seriously, to stand out for my leadership abilities, rather than my huge stomach. I also wanted a new job. I wanted to work in management development. I wanted to teach and train and speak and write professionally.

Beginning with the end in mind, is the first thing I had to do. I had to visualize my future self, being as specific as possible about how I wanted to look, and feel and act, and what I wanted to do and where I wanted to live. I wrote down my goals and referred to them often.

**Be the type of person who decides to do more than just dream big. The type of person who takes the time to visualize their future; instead of the type that just takes it as it comes. The type who decide who and where you want to be in five years. The type of person who begins with the end in mind.

2. PICK A START DATE

Sometimes I would catch a glimpse of myself in a mirror and be completely disgusted by the reflection, and sometimes I would catch someone else looking at me with an expression of disbelief, disgust and my favorite... anger; as if I was forcing them to carry the extra 150lbs. In either case, my face would burn with embarrassment, and I would get so mad at myself that I would scream.

"That's it! I've had it!" And then I would vow to get back on the wagon. "Starting tomorrow I am going to stop eating like an asshole!" I promised. And I meant it... every time.

Then tomorrow would come and I'd be completely unprepared. I wouldn't have a plan, or have the right foods in the house, or even know what the right foods were. The only thing I did have was the burning embarrassment from the day before. So I'd skip breakfast, thinking I would find a healthy alternative to the waffles, eggs, toast and bacon I normally had. Of course, by the time I left the house I would be starving, still unsure what I was supposed to be eating or where it is I was going to get it. Soon my embarrassment would turn into despair. Hungry and frustrated, I would push the rearview mirror up, blocking my own reflection and pull into the nearest fast food restaurant and start eat away my feelings; until next time.

Success finally came when I learned the value of picking a start date. Picking a start date is goal setting 101. Believe me, I know what it is like to get so frustrated that you want to throw yourself head first into whatever diet you are the most familiar with. I know what it is like to want to make big changes, to wake up and just be a different person, but trust me, if you want to have success in anything, especially losing weight, you need to give yourself some time to plan... and that begins with a start date.

A few points about picking a start date:

1. Pick a date that is at least two weeks away from right now. (Yes. Right now. Why else did you buy this book if you are not ready to get back on the wagon?).

2. Do not wait more than four weeks to start. (It is hard to stay focused and motivated beyond four weeks–Use this time to finish reading this book and getting yourself prepared).

3. Start this new adventure on a Friday (See Rule #3)

**Be the type of person who doesn't start something without a plan. The type of person who chooses a start date, is prepared, and sets themselves up to win. I know you're excited. That you are sick and tired of being sick and tired, but trust me; to succeed, you need a plan.

3. START ON FRIDAY

We always start new things on Mondays; a new job, a new workout routine, a new diet... It is the beginning of a new week after all, and starting something new on a Monday seemed reasonable; normal. It is like a new beginning. The problem with starting a diet on Monday, however, is that we need get through a Saturday and Sunday first.

I don't know what it is about Saturdays and Sundays; maybe it's because I have more time and flexibility to think about, and travel to, all the unhealthy food places I've been craving. Either way, I always eat way too much. Add the idea that I'm starting a new diet on Monday, and you'd think I was committing to never eating again.

I would have a fast food breakfast, a Chinese buffet lunch and then a dinner filled with pizza, wings, milkshakes, ice cream, and cake. I would eat so much that I'd be sick and could barely move.

"But this REALLY is the last time," I would tell myself; but it never was.

Overeating the night before I started a diet always set me up for failure. Most of us are addicted to sugar, and overloading the night before increases our cravings, making it harder for us to avoid them the next day.

I needed to break that cycle and so do you. You will have more success if you start on a Friday.

**Be the type of person who doesn't give yourself a weekend of overeating before you start your diet.

4. CHOOSE A PLAN

It doesn't matter if you are going to follow Weight Watchers (like me), or the Paleo Diet, or South Beach, or Atkins, or simply want to follow a calorie counting app on your phone. The most important thing is that you find a plan that is going to work for you – the best one is the one that closely resembles your current eating habits.

I travel a lot for work and eat out nearly three meals a day, five days a week. I had to find a plan that I could (easily) use in a grocery store, as well as in a restaurant.

If you are home every night, and you bring lunch to work every day, choose a plan that is better suited for that scenario. There are a lot of meal plans that have you prep all your meals for the whole week on Sundays, for example.

I would also caution you about extreme dieting – that is, choosing a diet that cuts out 90% of the foods you are currently eating. An all protein diet is easier for some people than it is for others. If your diet consists of a lot of carbs, going all protein may not be the best choice.

**Be the type of person who chooses the diet plan that mostly resembles your current habits. The type that understands making small adjustments in the beginning will give you bigger successes in the end.

5. LEARN EVERYTHING YOU CAN

I remember getting to chapter 11 in Dr. Atkins book and reading "First of all, let me welcome those of you who are starting the book at this point," (p. 121). I remember shaking my head in disbelief. I would have never thought of skipping ahead to chapter 11; to where the diets instructions started. For me, I always started on page one. Of course, I didn't always make it to chapter 11 before I had lost interest... so perhaps those people were on to something.

Here's the thing. If you are serious about losing the weight, about changing your life, about no longer wanting to be called the "Bigger Sister" or "Bigger Brother," then take the time to read, watch, study, plan, discuss, and learn everything you can about the diet plan you have chosen. Before you start.

Adventures in Dietland is a game millions of people play and only a handful win. Want to win? Then do your homework. Do whatever it takes to get as familiar with the diet plan you are choosing as you can.

The truth is, you are going to be dealing with a lot when you diet; and throwing in a difficult learning curve on how to use your new fancy app, while your struggling to resist donuts, just adds to your stress. Stress that you don't need.

**Be the type of person who does their homework. The type of person who no longer half-asses their diet, their eating plans... their life.

6. DO THE MATH

If you have been dieting for any length of time, you have probably heard the phrase: "Dieting is nothing more than the mathematical equation of calories in and calories out." While this is true, it took me a while to figure out what that mathematical equation looked like and how I could use it.

Consider this:

To maintain a weight of 350lbs (at 6' tall) I needed to eat 3,473 calories a day. I took that number and divided it by three, (3,473/3) and came up with 1,158 calories per meal.

Using Weight Watchers, at 350lbs, I was given 63 Points a day to eat. Dividing those Points up, meant that I had 21 Points per meal. Of course, we are not here to maintain 350lbs. We are here to lose weight.

At first, I tried to calculate how much I wanted to weigh (200lbs) and then figured out how many calories or Points I would need to eat at that level, (2,537 calories or 40 Points). I failed every time I tried it this way.

The truth is, you should reduce the amount you eat slowly. If you weigh 350lbs, calculate how many calories (or Points) you need to eat to weight ten pounds less, say 340lbs. At 340lbs I need to eat 3,410 calories or 61 Points. Reducing your caloric intake by 63 calories, or a couple of Points, is easier to accomplish – giving you much better results.

Do the math: To be successful, you will need to know what your numbers are, how you get those numbers and what it means per day and per meal.

**Be the type of person who does the math. The type of person who takes the time to calculate exactly how many carbs or protein, or calories or Points, that you need, for every meal.

7. TRACK YOUR FOOD

Do you believe in magic?

Try tracking what you spend, or how many pushups you can do in a single setting or your test scores, or how much data you (or your kids) use on a daily basis. If you do, you will notice something remarkable. You will begin to spend less. You will do more pushups, have higher test scores and gain more control over your data plan; even if you didn't intend too. It's magic.

This same "magic" happens when you keep track of what you eat. The more you track, the less you will eat. Tracking what you eat, every meal, every day, is "The Key" to losing weight. It is the difference maker between success and failure. Being fat or being thin. It is all about tracking.

When I suggest to people that they should use a program like Weight Watchers, I get the same response. No one wants to count Points. Here's the thing. It doesn't matter if you are counting calories, or carbs, or Points, you must count, or it won't work. It is that simple. The best part is that there are all kinds of apps and calculators and online tools that make counting calories, or carbs or WW Points, extremely easy.

The problem with easy, of course, is everything that is easy to do, is just as easy not to do. I know it might take you a couple of times to read that sentence to get what I'm saying, so I am going to repeat it. "The problem with easy is, everything that is easy to do, is just as easy, not to do."

"But tracking isn't easy." I can see you shaking your head in disbelief, as if I have just gone off the deep end. But let's be honest; being fat isn't easy either. It is not fun, it is not productive, it is not flattering, it isn't healthy, and it takes a ton of work to maintain such a big ass. Trust me, I know!

Do you want to lose that ass of yours? Then start keeping track of all the food you eat. It is that simple.

**Be the type of person who tracks everything you eat.

8. GET TO KNOW YOUR DOCTOR

My doctor's name is Lynn. For the longest time, she was Dr. So, and So. And Dr. So, and So and I did not have the best relationship. We were both polite and cordial, of course, but our appointments were always contentious. She would look at my weight, blood pressure, and the results from my latest lab work and ask me how I was feeling. Embarrassed I would lie and tell her I was great. She would nod, tight lipped, and reread the results, as if she missed something. She hadn't.

Every time I saw her I was heavier than I was the last time. My blood pressure was worse, my cholesterol levels where troubling and I barely fit in the patient chair in her office. And every time she would bring up one of these issues, I would get defensive.

After years of this, and I mean years... I finally had had enough.

"Lynn," I said, catching her off guard. "Can I call you Lynn?" She nodded and took in some air. Then she looked at me, waiting. It had been four months since our last appointment. "Lynn," I said. I could feel my face start to burn red with embarrassment. I was finally going to come clean. "I'm a mess," I said. I struggled with the words. "And I've got to figure this out." She held my gaze for a minute and then smiled. She reached out and put her hand on my mine.

"We can figure this out Ralph… we can turn this around. It's not too late."

Ever since I have been on a first name basis with my Doctor, I have stopped lying, stopped making excuses and started listening to what she had to say. I used to see her every four to six months and try to tell her everything was okay. Now our scheduled check-ups are every eighteen months, because I am okay. I'm better than okay. I'm doing great. And it all started the day I got to know my doctor.

**Be the type of person that is on a first name basis with your doctor. Be the type of person that is so open and honest about you, and how you are feeling, that they know everything, and can help.

9. GET ON THE SCALE

"It's not going to bite," the nurse said when I hesitated.

"I wouldn't be so sure," I said. I had only one foot on the scale as if I was trying to get used to the pool temperature before diving in.

"Come on. Come on. I haven't got all day," she said.

Getting on the scale is never easy. Even today, with all my weight loss success, I still hesitate. I still cringe. I still exhale as much as I can, just in case the extra air in my lungs is the difference between .9 and 1 pound.

Getting on a scale is one of those necessary evils. No one wants to "know" how much they weigh. Especially those of us who are battling weight gain, or worse, have had some success in losing weight and then fell off the proverbial "wagon" and gained it all back... and more. However, it is the only way to begin this process. You need to have a starting point; a starting weight. Then, what do you do with that number? You track it, of course.

TIP 9.5 BUY YOUR OWN SCALE

Scales fluctuate. My scale at home is always a couple of pounds different from the scale at the doctor, and worse, at Weight Watchers – though sometimes it works to my benefit.

More than buying your own scale, using the same scale, at the same time, on the same day of the week, is going to give you the most accurate results. It doesn't matter if you buy your own scale or use someone else's. Pick one, and stick to it.

**Be the type of person that gets on the scale, every week, no matter what. It doesn't matter if you are having a good week, or a bad week. Just like tracking your food, there is magic in keeping track of your weight.

10. TOUGHEN UP

There is a diet book called "Get Tough or Die Fat," by Steve Siebold (2010). I haven't read it, but I know who Steve is, he is a Mental Toughness guru, and the title has always stuck with me. Get tough or die fat. What a horrible situation to be in, but that is where I found myself. And that is where you, if you are reading this book, are finding yourself.

Beyond tracking and doing the math and setting up food zones, and going to the doctor and getting new friends, truthfully... I had to toughen up. I had to take control of my mind – of that little bastard that is constantly telling me that dieting is too hard, that I need to sleep more, that running is bad for me, that I'm getting too thin, and worst of all that, "We are all going to die of something..." so why bother with anything.

It's easy to read through these tips and see how some make sense for you, while others don't. None of them matter, however, if you are not going to put your foot down and toughen up. You are not going to die from hunger pains. At 260lbs, was not getting too skinny, and (for most of us) you do not need to have surgery. You need to toughen up.

Jump, Scream, Curse! (Rule #28); start putting yourself first (Rule #30); learn to celebrate without food, and always... regardless of what you eat, keep track (Rule #7).

**Be the type of person who would rather throw themselves on the floor, four-year-old style – pitching a fit, than to give in. The type of person who talks to themselves. The type of person who is willing to suffer short term, so they can live the life of their dreams in the long term. It's worth it... You my friend, are worth it. Toughen up.

11. QUIT THE GYM

The number is in the thousands. Thousands of dollars in gym memberships that I never used. $10, $25, even $150 a month, wasted on a gym that I never attended.

I always had the best intentions. I'd usually join the gym some-time in January, thinking that this was it. This was the year that I was going to make going to the gym a priority. And I would... for a week... sometimes two weeks... and then something would happen.

As I said in the beginning, I grew up fat. I never learned how to exercise or lift weights or stretch. So when I went to the gym I would always overdo it, and get hurt, every time. Then I would take a couple of days off, which would then turn into a couple of years...

The worst part about paying for a gym that you don't use, is the guilt you feel. It seems ridiculous and completely unintentional, but if I didn't go to the gym to work out, then I wouldn't work out at all.

I cannot tell you how many nights I went to bed, with the inten-tion of going to the gym in the morning – only to wake up full of excuses on why I didn't have time to drive all the way to the gym, pick up heavy stuff, then put it down – repeat a bunch of times and then what... Shower there? Should I bring my work clothes with me and then go to work? Or should I just go home and shower? Do I have time to go there, work out and then go home, before going to work?

Of course, I didn't. So I wouldn't. I never went to the gym and, because I was paying for it, never worked out unless I was at the gym.

Finally, sick and tired of being sick and tired, I quit paying for a gym membership I didn't use and started walking. Every morning, regardless of the weather, or how I was feeling, or how much time I had, I went for a walk. Some days I had fifteen minutes, other days I had an hour. Every day, I walked.

**Be the type of person who stops using your gym membership as an excuse not to exercise. Be the type of person who quits the gym, buys a pair of running shoes, walks out the front door of their house and takes a right or a left, every day. Be the type of person who doesn't need to go somewhere to work out.

12. DO THE DISHES

When I smoked cigarettes, one of my favorite times to light up was right after a meal. It didn't matter if it was breakfast, lunch or dinner. For some reason, I craved cigarettes more after I ate, than at any other time. During the smoking cessation class I took to quit, I found out that nearly everyone who smokes likes to light up after they eat.

"Do the dishes," the instructor told us. "Once you are done eating, get up and start to clean up. Put your hands in warm soapy water. Do you know how hard it is to smoke with your hands in warm soapy water?"

This little piece of advice worked. The whole idea of not sitting around – especially during those trigger times, when you most likely over eat, or smoke, or drink – is key to how I have been able to stop smoking, drinking and over eating.

**Be the type of person who has the cleanest kitchen in the

neighborhood. The type of person who, as soon as they are done eating, jumps up and sticks their hands in a warm soapy water, instead of more food.

13. PEE IN THE WOODS

They would eyeball me as I walked in. "The bathroom is for customers only," they'd want to say but don't. Doesn't matter. I'd feel guilty anyway and I was never shy about grabbing some fries, or maybe some chicken, or a milk shake.

I'd like to say I only did this occasionally, but the truth is, I stopped at a fast food restaurant every time I had to pee – which considering how much time I spend on the road, is a lot; and by "a lot" I mean a few times a day. Every time, I would go in, use the bathroom and walk out with a bag full of food. A burger, some fries, maybe a milk shake. It was always something. But it didn't stop there. It wasn't just fast food places. It was convenience stores and coffee shops and grocery stores. Everywhere I stopped to pee, I would buy food.

Finally, reluctantly, I decided I was no longer going to buy any food from any of these places, just because I needed to use the bathroom. I was no longer going to feel guilty. And I meant it. Until I walked in and smelled the pizza, or the French fries, or saw all the delicious donuts...

Maybe it isn't guilt I was feeling. Maybe I just can't be trusted around fast food and instead of facing that, I had developed an excuse. I mean. They are letting me use their bathroom. The least I could do was buy something. Not anymore.

**Be the type of person who would rather pull off the side of the road and pee in the woods, than the type that is constantly putting themselves in a situation that they clearly cannot handle.

14. BURN YOUR FAT CLOTHES

This is a story about the same thing happening to me, over and over again. Maybe you can relate.

I would finally have enough of all the overeating, of being the fat guy. I would put my foot down. Enough is enough, I would tell myself. Then, I would work hard. I would follow a diet perfectly and have some great success. I mean, big success. Going down a full shirt size or two, type of success. Going from a 48-inch waste to a 44-inch waste, kind of success.

As I lost the weight I would go to my closet and begin to pull out my "Skinny-er" clothes, allowing my fat clothes to pile up on the floor. Usually in a corner somewhere. After a few weeks, my wife would yell at me about all the clothes on the floor and I would pick them up, and put them in garbage bags next to the door.

I always intended to throw them in my car and drop them off in one of those Goodwill drop boxes. Key word, "intended." In truth, they never left their spot by the door... until I started to gain again. Soon I would be head first into the bag trying to find a pair of pants that I didn't have to hold my breath while wearing.

Before long, my "Skinny-er" clothes would make their way back into my closet, or the very bottom drawer of my dresser and I'd be wearing all of my fat clothes again. Then I read a book called "Fat Guy Friday," by Craig Beck.

In his book, he described going through the same thing I was going through. Having some success; going down a couple of pant sizes; only to go back up. Finally, he figured out, holding on to the fat clothes was allowing him to continue this yo yo'ing. So he set out to destroy every piece of clothing that was too big for him. Every time he went down a size, everything that was a size up, he destroyed and threw away. It works.

To this day, I don't have any shirts that are 2X, or even 1X. That's crazy. You know why I don't have anything that's 1X or 2X or 3X? Because I will never be that heavy again. It's purely psychological.

**Be the type of person who is so committed to losing weight, to changing your life, that you destroy every piece of clothing that is too big for you right now. Literally. This book can wait. Go to your closet and grab everything that is too big for you. Then start tearing them up. Cut them up. Roll around in the mud with them. Burn them. Kill your fat clothes... and then throw them away.

15. WASTE YOUR FOOD

Growing up, we were never allowed to leave the dinner table until we finished eating. When we'd cry and moan, mom would tell us about these poor children in Africa who were, at that very moment, going without dinner because there wasn't enough food.

It's funny how I took that habit into adulthood. I eat everything on my plate, every chip that's in the bag, every cookie that is in the box, every M&M that comes in the large package... I never wasted food.

I remember the first time that I did waste food; intentionally. I was walking around a grocery store looking for a snack. It was after lunch, but way before dinner, so I didn't have a lot of points to waste on a snack. I was craving humus and crackers. I took out my phone, and scanned the bar code with my WW app.

Humus was 2 points per serving, however, the package contained 3 servings. I knew myself well enough to know that if I got into my car with 3 servings of humus, I would eat all three servings. That is when I got the idea. The idea to waste my food. Then I went looking for crackers. Plain rice crackers contain the least amount of points (2 per serving). But again, the box contained 6 servings.

Just outside of the grocery store, right next to the door, there was a garbage can. I stopped, opened the box of crackers, counted out 8 crackers (one serving), and threw the rest away. I did the same thing with the humus. I divided it up into thirds, and then scooped two-thirds into the trash.

I cannot tell you how great it felt and how wonderful it works. I'm the type of person who cleans my plate, who eats all the chips, who can't stop picking at something if it is beside me in the car, even though I've had enough.

**Be the type of person who is willing to waste their food. The type of person who knows how much they should be eating and throws the rest away.

16. DOGGY BAGS ARE FOR DOGS

I wouldn't just take a doggy bag home from a restaurant, I would intentionally order more than I could eat, (which is a lot), just so I could take home a doggy bag. Here's the thing, I've never owned a dog.

There are some that suggest you ask for a "To Go Box" right when you order. That way, you can split your meal in half, before you start eating. Once the food is in the "To Go Box" it is out of sight and out of mind and you will only eat what you are supposed to. Then, you get to take the other half of the meal home to have at another time.

It is a perfect strategy that works for many people. However, it didn't work for me. I am an over eater. Meaning, I couldn't pack a lunch without getting into it on my way in to work. If it was beside me, then I would eat it. Same thing with a doggy bag. Instead of eating at the restaurant, I would eat it in the car on the way home from the restaurant.

**Be the type of person that asks for a "To Go Box" before you start eating, so you can make up your very own doggy bag – if you have a dog that you are truly going to give it to. Otherwise, be the type of person who leaves restaurant food at the restaurant – even if that means, half your meal, (or toss it in the trash on your way out (Rule #15)).

17. TALK TO YOURSELF

How can you tell if you are hungry or if you are just bored? How can you tell if you are full or not? How do you stop yourself from cheating? How do you stay on track? How do you overcome cravings? How do you quiet down the voices in your head that are constantly making excuses for you?

Start talking to yourself. Start paying attention. Start assessing, and planning, rather than reacting and giving in.

It has taken me a long time to figure out how much food is enough food for me. I cannot rely on my stomach, it lies to me. I cannot rely on my taste buds, they lie to me too. I have to rely on my eyeballs, first, and then my patience.

I have to measure out my food (which is always a smaller portion than I want), eat slowly, deliberately, and then suffer the voices in my head, the voices that are reminding me how good the meal was, and that there is more in the kitchen, or if I'm out at a restaurant, that it wasn't quite enough and the waitress would love to show me a dessert menu.

"You are fine Ralph," I say. "You don't need any more food. You've had enough. Be strong. Be patient." And then sometimes I start singing randomly... anything to distract that voice in my head.

We all talk to ourselves. We all have an inner voice that is constantly narrating our lives to us. Telling us we are hungry when we are not. Telling us we deserve dessert or an extra serving or another slice. Talk over that voice. Be louder, stronger, bolder.

**Be the type of person who talks to themselves. The type of person that no longer goes along with the same narrative that has played over and over again, telling you how weak you are. Be louder, stronger, bolder.

18. SET AN ALARM

I never have a problem eating breakfast or lunch. Like clockwork, I eat breakfast and lunch at the same times, every day. Dinner, however. Dinner has always been a struggle. Sometimes I work too late. Sometimes I'm waiting for a friend to eat with me. And then there are times that I eat too soon.

Either way, dinner has always been my nemesis. It is the time of day that I eat the most food, and the time I am most likely to overeat. Additionally, it is also the meal that I am generally the least prepared for.

This craziness went on forever... until finally, I realized that I had this nifty little thing called a smart phone in my pocket; and it had an alarm. An alarm that I was using for everything else, so why not set it to remind myself to eat dinner?

I got it wrong the first few times I tried to do it, setting it for when I wanted to eat, rather than when I should start thinking and planning on eating; which, it turns out, is the key. Now, I have an alarm set for 5pm every day. I intend to eat by 5:30 or 6pm. By setting the alarm 30 minutes early (5pm) it gives me time to assess where I am, decide what I am eating, and plan my meal before hunger sets in and I go and grab the closest, easiest, and (usually) the unhealthiest thing that I can find.

**Be the type of person who sets an alarm. The type of person who gives themselves time to plan their meals, before hunger sets in and you make bad decisions.

19. GET NEW FRIENDS

Before you skip this tip, hear me out. If you are serious about losing weight – the kind of weight that you have to lose in order to change your life (like me) – then you probably already know what I am about to say. You cannot surround yourself with people that stuff themselves with quarts of ice cream, bags of chips and boxes of cookies while sitting on the couch watching television for hours each night, and expect to change. The truth is, we are the total sum of who we surround ourselves with.

When I quit drinking, and smoking, and eating like an asshole, I had to stop hanging out with my friends who drank and smoked and ate like assholes. Have you ever tried to quit smoking while riding back and forth to work with someone who constantly smokes? Or go to a bar and not drink alcohol? Have you ever gone to an all you can eat Chinese buffet, and had just one small plate of vegetables?

No. The truth is, if you were trying to quit drinking alcohol, you wouldn't go to a bar. It's the same thing with food – and your friends.

**Be the type of person who tries to get all of their friends to live healthier life styles through diet and exercise. The type of person who is supportive and understanding if their friends don't want to (it may not be their time). Be the type of person who is able to recognize the difference. The type of person who is willing to move on, to find new friends, to separate themselves from temptation.

20. THINK ABOUT PUSHUPS

If you don't know who Matthew McConaughey is, then Google him. He's an actor who has made some amazing films.

In 2012 he starred in a movie called Magic Mike (Steven Soderbergh, Warner Bros.). The movie is about an older male stripper, teaching a younger male stripper how to live the life of a male stripper. I know it sounds confusing, and I'm over simplifying, but it's not relevant.

The point I want to make is Mathew McConaughey had to get into incredible shape for this movie. And by incredible shape, I mean, the zero-body-fat, six-pack-abs, kind of shape. During an interview, he was asked to identify the one thing that he did every day to get in such great shape.

"Every time I thought of pushups," he said. "I did pushups."

Imagine that. Imagine if you were so dedicated to having an amazing body, to being in shape, to looking good, to feeling good, that every time you thought about pushups; you did pushups. You don't have to do a lot. If you can only do one pushup, then do one pushup. If you can do ten, then do ten.

**Be the type of person that is so dedicated to living a healthy life style that you are willing to take on this challenge. Pushups not your thing? Then try it with squats, or jumping jacks, or lunges. Be the type of person that is active – all the time.

21. THROW AWAY YOUR MICROWAVE

If you remember from the beginning of this book–the hero's journey as I like to refer to it – you should recall that my family got our first microwave when I was about 15 or 16 years old, and it basically took away both my patience with food, and my need to learn how to cook and prepare meals.

I remember buying my first microwave for my first apartment. Then my second, and third. When I bought a house, I had a microwave permanently installed above the stove. Everything revolved around that microwave. Everything I bought was microwavable, convenient and easy.

Finally, after seeing the microwave for what it really was (a problem) I vowed to stop using it. Instead, I decided that I was going to learn how to cook; using actual pots and pans – old school style. You may not believe this but an amazing thing started to happen. The food came out better. Looked better. Tasted better. I started to shop more and spend more time in a grocery store looking at ingredients and trying challenging recipes. I began to cook.

The more I cooked and looked at recipes and prepared, chopped, blended, filet, scrubbed, blanched, baked, seared, broiled, and simmered, the more I learned and the better I ate.

Throw away your microwave.

**Be the type of person who cooks, from scratch. Start with just one meal a day. Then two. Then all three. Be the type of person who makes time to cook, to eat right, to prepare. The type of person who is willing to learn everything you can about one of the most important thing in your life, the food you eat.

22. STOP LISTENING TO YOUR BODY

"Hello everyone, my name is Ralph Peterson and my body is a big fat liar." I feel like I should be starting this tip as if I am attending an AA meeting for the first time; that is, as both an introduction and a confession. The problem with my body being a big fat liar, is how long I have listened to it... even though I knew better.

To be clear, my body isn't just misinformed or misunderstood. It blatantly, out and out lies to me. It tells me I'm hungry when I'm not hungry. It tells me I didn't have enough food when I clearly did. It tells me it's okay to sit longer or lay in bed and sleep extra. It tells me I've exercised enough when I clearly haven't. Or worse, it tries to remind me that I did work out this morning and so going for seconds, or buying those M&M's or having a cookie is more than okay, it's deserved.

If you ask my body, it will tell you that it knows exactly what I need to eat, how much and when. Don't believe it.

I know what I need. I need a lean protein, a good carb and a vegetable. Throw in some fruit, and that's it. I don't need to go for seconds, I don't need a dinner roll or deserve dessert because I am going without butter. I needed to stop listening to my body.

**Be the type of person who stops listening to their body. The type of person who has done the math, figured out the calculations, measures, weighs and puts only what their body needs on their plate, despite what your body is saying.

23. DIET LIKE IT IS YOUR JOB

I was channel surfing one day and came across one of those work out video infomercials for perfect abs. The commercial featured a guy and a girl and a piece of equipment that "If you used every day, would give you perfect looking abs." Of course, both the guy and the girl in the video had perfect abs. It got me thinking.

What if your weight loss goals, what if being thin, what if having six-pack abs, and being in the best shape possible, was your job? I mean, for the guy and girl in this commercial – it is their job.

What would it look like if you ate right and exercised for a living. What would you do? How often would you work out? What exercise would you do? What would you eat? How much would you eat? When would you eat? What would your job routine look like?

Right now, I get to work at 8am. I go to my office. I check and respond to emails, look at what I have coming up for the rest of the day. I usually have a conference call at 9am to discuss projects we are working on. I take lunch at noon, and on and on.

What if I wrote that same type of job routine for leading a healthy life.

I get up at 5:30am and drink a tall glass of room temperature water. I put on my running shoes and head out for a walk or a run by 6am. At 7am, I shower. At 7:30 I make breakfast: One cup of plain oatmeal with a banana and three egg whites scrambled. I live close to my office, so I don't have to leave my house until 7:50am. I arrive at work at 8am. At 10am I am going to be a bit hungry, and so I brought an apple and a tablespoon of peanut butter as a snack. Continue to work. At noon, I am going to eat the lunch I brought and then go for a walk around the block with the remaining 15 minutes I have before I have to get back to work... and on and on and on.

**Be the type of person who treats their diet and their health, like it is your job. Like you get paid to do it. Paid to eat right and exercise, every meal; every day. In the end, you do. We all do. We all get paid based on our abilities to think and move and act and work and lead. We all get paid to take care of ourselves.

24. CREATE A SENSE OF URGENCY

When I woke up fat, on April 25 2013, I had a lot of reasons to be scared. Most of all, I was scared of time. Had I run out of time? Did I wake up fat – too late? Had I already caused irreversible damage to myself, from years of binge drinking and overeating?

When my dad was diagnosed with emphysema he quit smoking cigarettes immediately – but it was too late. The damage had already been done. I remember him explaining to me. That quitting smoking was more about the quality of his remaining life, than about curing anything. Getting emphysema was a death sentence for my dad. There was nothing he could do about it. He quit too late.

We only have this one life. This one heart and one set of lungs. Don't wait until you finish this book, or until you eat all the junk food in your house, or wait until you can talk your significant other into dieting with you... you have to start right now. It's urgent.

**Be the type of person who is in a rush to get healthy. The type of person who puts their own health above everything, and everyone in their life.

25. STALK THIN PEOPLE

We were in a large exhibit hall, maybe fifty vendors, with individual booths trying to get people to stop and ask us about our products. Around 4pm, caterers began setting up for a cocktail party that was to begin at 5pm in the same room.

As my luck would have it, they put the finger food station right in front of my booth. It was made up of three six-foot-long tables full of all kinds of vegetables, and cheeses (soft and hard), and crackers, peperoni, cut up fruit, bread and more spreads and dipping sauces than you would have expected.

It didn't take too long for a couple of us to start reaching in and helping ourselves. I went for the cheese and peperoni. The guy beside me went for the bread, and the lady across from us, very thin and very pretty, reached in and grabbed a cherry tomato. Just one.

I wanted to say something to her. To be funny and sarcastic, but I didn't. I just watched her. Five minutes went by – I'm not exaggerating – five whole minutes before she reached in again, this time grabbing a slice of red pepper. Just one.

I remember this other time I was at breakfast; it was a whole group of us from work. I watched a coworker, this tiny lady, eat a half, of a half of an English muffin. That's it. That's all she ate. For breakfast. One half, of one half of an English muffin. That is when I started stalking thin people.

That is when I realized one of the best ways for me to learn how much food to eat, was to find someone that I wanted to look like – and watch what they ate. How much they ate and what they did between bites of food. How long did it take them to eat? Did they stop when they were full or when the food was gone? Did they go for seconds? I know this might sound creepy, but trust me... you can learn a lot by stalking thin people.

**Be the type of person who watches what other people eat. The type of person who, when you find someone who looks like the person you want to look like, pays attention to what that person is eating, how much, and how often. Be the type of person who stalks thin people.

26. STOP SUPPORTING THE TROOPS

We have all seen them, the boxes of candy, the buckets of cookie dough, the dozens of frozen pizzas (the, assemble yourself kind) and of course the cookies... lots and lots of cookies. I have always been a sucker for charity; for supporting the troops. Well, as long as those charities involve candy, cookie dough, pizza and / or cookies.

It's funny, in a ridiculous sort of way. I mean, I have never gone to the market and thought, "You know what I need... a big bucket of cookie dough, or a twelve pack of assemble your own pizzas...," but if a kid came knocking on my front door with a big smile and an order form, I wouldn't hesitate. It's for charity after all; I'm supporting the troops.

Of course, the charity in question, takes all the proceeds they make from cookie sales and feeds the poor, supports education, and helps kids learn valuable life skills. The whole time, I'm sitting on the couch, using my newly arrived bucket of cookie dough to make thin mint sandwiches while I'm waiting for the pizza to finish cooking.

"But hey, I'm a giver," I reason. "I like to help out." At least that is what I tell myself when I was contemplating the number of boxes I should be ordering. "Is three of each going to be enough, or should I make it an even five?"

The truth is, I shouldn't have been ordering any. I was one hundred and fifty pounds' overweight. Only a hand full of cookies away from developing type II diabetes and my cholesterol was so high I had to be on medication for it. Yet, despite all of this, I couldn't control myself. If there are cookies in my house (even today), I will eat them. The same is true for candy, cookie dough, pizza, cake, muffins, ice cream, pretzels, chips, nuts, popcorn..., you name it. If it's within reach, I'm reaching.

Finally, I had to stop supporting the troops. I had to stop fooling myself into believing their charity was more important than my waistline, my health and my happiness. I had to become the type of person who doesn't buy junk food, regardless of who is selling it.

**Be the type of person who is charitable, who does support the troops, but doesn't do it by buying junk food.

27. STAY OFF THE GRASS

We've all seen them. Dirt paths cut across, otherwise, perfectly manicured lawns. Most commonly you can see these at universities. In fact, it is so common and such a big eyesore, many universities have decided to forgo the traditional box shaped lawns, with uniform sidewalks, and instead let the students decide the route to their classes. Only then, after a well-worn path is established, does the university put in sidewalks.

When I was in the Marine Corps the only time I was ever allowed to walk on the grass was when I was exercising. "If you are not in PT gear and doing calisthenics, then stay off the grass." I can still hear the gruff voice of my First Sargent, screaming that senti-ment to anyone and everyone who he caught taking a short cut. And that is what walking on the grass is; a short cut.

I know that this may seem like a very small, insignificant detail, but this was a way of life for me. I took shortcuts everywhere I could. I took the elevator up one flight. I bought easy to prepare, done in 60 seconds, microwavable food. I always used a drive thru or parked as close as I could to the store and the only time I would stay off the grass was when it was raining, snowing or if the side-walk happened to be the shortest route.

Taking short cuts, miss managing my time, not being prepared, and running late, played a huge part as to how I woke up fat.

**Be the type of person who no longer takes shortcuts. The type of person who doesn't use a drive thru, or parks so close to the store that you almost need a handicap sign. Be the type of person who doesn't use a microwave and, for the love of God, stays off the grass.

28. JUMP, SCREAM, CURSE!

One of my biggest challenges was (and continues to be), how to deal with "Phantom" hunger pains. I say they are "Phantom," because, well... let's be honest, I have never TRULY gone hungry. Then I stubbed my toe.

"Ouch, ouch, ouch...," I yelled as I jumped around. Then I cursed, held my foot up and squeezed my eyes shut, waiting for the searing pain to go away. After a few more minutes of jumping around, yelling and cursing, the pain finally began to subside; and that's when I began to think about hunger pains.

I know it may sound silly, heck most of these tips probably sound silly, but trust me, it works. The next time it is 11am and lunch is at 12pm and you start feeling like you are not going to make it until noon, start jumping around. If you are in a place where you can yell and curse, I suggest you do that too. If not, grit your teeth and jump around.

**Be the type of person who is willing to do anything and everything to distract yourself from eating, when it isn't time to eat. Be the type of person who would rather make a fool out of themselves by jumping, yelling and cursing, than the type of person who is too embarrassed to jump, yell and curse, and instead find themselves giving in, eating early and gaining weight.

29. STOP TREATING EVERY MEAL AS IF IT IS YOUR LAST

I eat out a lot... nearly all three meals a day, every day. I travel a lot for work, and other than the free continental breakfast most hotels offer, I am usually at a restaurant for lunch and dinner. Here's the thing. Going out to eat, as much as I do, you tend to want to try all the decadent items on the menu. Everything looks and sounds amazing and for the longest time, I ordered on a whim. Whatever sounded good, I ordered. Sweet, savory, breaded, cheesy, unique, homemade, full flavor, real buttery deliciousness... you name it... I ordered it.

I have an affinity for Tator Tots and cheeseburgers and ice cream and mayonnaise and soda and donuts and fast food, fried food, food dipped in sugar, and food dipped in chocolate, or cooked in butter, pizza and chicken wings. You name it, I love it. I cannot tell you how many meals I have had that included almost every one of these items at one time. No wonder I weighed 350lbs! I treated every meal as if it were my last meal on earth. As if my life could end at any given moment and I didn't want to go without first trying a cheeseburger that uses two jelly filled donuts as the bun. "You're going to die of something..."

The truth, ironically, is that the more I ate, as if it were my last meal on earth, the more likely it was becoming that it would be. I was literally killing myself with the food choices I was making.

In Community College, I had to take Basic Biology twice – due to my lack of sufficient study habits – The good thing about taking the same class twice is that everything I learned the first time, I was able to master the second time. One of these concepts was on feeding cells. "That is all eating is, at its most basic biological level, feeding cells," the professor said, for the second time.

I think about that all the time now. Every time I am eating. "I'm just feeding cells," I remind myself. "And my mitochondrion, doesn't need a donut to be active."

**Be the type of person who doesn't treat every meal as if it is your last. Be the type of person who sticks to their plan, makes good choices and when you go out, eats like you want to keep living.

30. PUT YOURSELF FIRST

When flying on an airplane, the flight attendants go through a brief safety overview. During that time, they show you how to buckle your seat belt, where the exits are, how to inflate your life vest and, "In the event of loss cabin pressure, oxygen masks will fall from the ceiling;" how to put on your mask.

"If you are traveling with small children, or someone who needs assistance," they say. "Put your own mask on first, before assisting others with theirs." What a great concept.

For many of us, it is our children or our spouses, or work, or school, or a combination of all four. Somehow, somewhere along the line, everyone and everything became more important than ourselves. For me, it was work.

I would start work the moment I woke up, and continue until I went to bed. There was always something to do, an email to respond to, a client to contact, a report to review and a place to go. I never took time for anything else. Note the word "took." When I first wrote this tip, I used the word "had," as in, "I never had time for anything else." But that is not true. I simply didn't take the time. I never put my own mask on first and I suffered the consequences.

You know what I am talking about... April 25th. That day that I woke up realizing that while I was busy making sure my "work" had its mask on, I was struggling to breath.

Put yourself first. Take time today, right now, to plan the rest of your day, and the rest of this week. You know what you need. You need to exercise and eat well, every day. Take the time to do both, before doing anything else for anyone else. Be selfish. It's worth it. You are worth it.

**Be the type of person who recognizes that they cannot continue to take care of others, without first taking care of themselves. The type of person that puts their health and wellbeing above everyone else's. Not out of spite or selfishness, but out of love and understanding. The type of person who puts their own mask on first.

31. PRE-GAME

When I was younger my friends and I would "Pre-Game" before we went out to our favorite hang-out, the bar. Pre-Gaming meant that we would drink, before we went out to drink.

The reason we did this is so that we wouldn't have to drink as much, (at the bar) to get drunk – because drinking at the bar is expensive. It is far cheaper to buy a case of beer, and split it with your friends at home, then it is to buy that same case of beer at the bar.

The same is true when shopping.

To be honest, I can't do it. I can go to the store. I can be ready with the list of foods I need for the week, and the coupons that I can use and all the cash in my pocket to pay for it all, but if I am hungry when I get there, the only thing I think about is finding something that I can eat, as quickly as possible.

I would be that person who helps himself to a few grapes, or opens a box of crackers, or a bag of chips, (and a diet cola) and walks around stuffing my face as I shop. Of course, if I'm already blowing my diet – eating Salt & Vinegar potato chips and drinking Diet Coke – I would start reaching for anything and everything that I was craving: cupcakes, candy, ice cream, maybe a donut or two...

Here's the thing, when I shop hungry I crave quick, easy, convenient foods, that normally have three times as many points (or calories) than I am supposed to have; which makes it so that I end up paying for the food twice. First I pay with cash and then I pay for it with my growing waste line. The latter being the most expensive.

**Be the type of person who pre-games before shopping. Schedule your shopping trip right after a meal. It is a great way of being active right after you eat, and it will help you stay away from impulsively buying (and craving) foods that you shouldn't have.

31.5 BONUS TIP: RUN—DON'T WALK, IN A GROCERY STORE.

Grocery stores have both the best or worst food on the planet. The problem I have with shopping, is that I would do just that. I would shop. I would walk down every aisle, look at every item, and end up buying a lot more stuff than I need. And I'm- not only talking about "bad for me" stuff. I would simply end up buying too much food. More food than I can eat, and certainly more than I need.

**Be the type of person who is on a mission, a mission to get in and out of the grocery store as fast as possible. Save the meandering, walking down every aisle, looking at everything, type of shopping for new (smaller) clothes.

32. STAY AWAY... FROM BUFFETS...

I want to tell you about the last time I went to an all-you-can-eat Chinese buffet with my dad. It was his treat. He loved Chinese food. I remember sitting there and watching him come back to the table with three plates full of food. I said, "You know you can keep going back up for more." He looked at me and then his three plates of food and smiled.

"Yeah," he said. "But I don't want to." I laughed and shook my head. Too funny.

You didn't need me to tell you that story. Just like you don't need me to tell you that my dad was heavy my whole life (and maybe his). Or that nearly everyone I know who eats at an all-you-can-eat Chinese buffet, regularly, is either heavy, or well on their way to being heavy.

The truth is, you really don't need me to say anything at all about this tip... So I won't.

**Be the type of person that stay's as far away from an all-you-can-eat buffet as you can, regardless of what kind of food is being served.

33. USE CHOPSTICKS

It was one of those life hack columns. The ones that give you tiny little tips that turn out to be extremely useful, like using Post-it notes to clean in between your keyboard, or peeling a banana from the bottom, or using "chopsticks" to eat Cheetos's, so that your fingers don't turn orange.

Chopsticks for Cheeto's? What a great idea... But I don't eat a lot of Cheetos. I do, however, eat a lot of popcorn. Especially movie popcorn. I tried it and you wouldn't believe what happened: I couldn't scarf down the popcorn, like I always did.

I was always the type of person who finishes their bag of popcorn before the movie starts. The kind of person who eat way more than my fair share of the popcorn. I want to say it is because I'm the youngest of four and have had to battle for such treats like popcorn; and maybe that is where it started, but not anymore. Now I'm filling my face full of popcorn by the fistful because I love it and I have very little control... until I started using chop sticks.

Now I use chopsticks on everything I can. I even bring them to the movies with me.

**Be the type of person who uses chopsticks to eat anything that you normally shovel in your face by the hand full. Potato chips, popcorn, almonds, grapes.... Whatever you eat... be the type of person who uses chopsticks; slows down, and enjoys every bite.

33.5 BONUS TIP

For those of you who, like me, didn't have the first clue how to use chop sticks, don't fret. Not knowing how to use chop sticks is going to be extremely helpful. It will slow you down even more... which is the point.

**Be the type of person who did what I did... I went to www. Youtube.com, watched a bunch of videos and practiced.

34. EAT ALONE

In the beginning, I was dieting alone and every time I ate with my friends, they always ordered the most decadent food items on the menu. It was tough. It is tough. Trying to eat healthy while everyone else at your table is ordering chicken wing appetizers and then following it up with cheese burgers and truffle fries.

The worst part, is none of them cared if I ordered and ate the same things they were having. But if I order a salad, or ask for a plain piece of chicken, the harassment never ends. I don't know if they are feeling bad about what they are eating, or if they are just looking for any reason to bust my chops, but it is difficult to eat healthy in front of people who are not eating healthy.

Drinking is the same way. No one understands, or likes the fact that I don't drink; especially when they are drinking. Everyone is constantly trying to get me to have "just one," drink with them.

Eat alone. This is probably one of the best pieces of advice I can give you. If you can't get new friends, stop eating with your old ones.

**Be the type of person who knows better than to eat with people who are not going to be supportive. The type of person who does not put themselves in situations where temptation is going to be too much to handle.

35. ACT LIKE A KID

Do you remember what it was like when you were five or six years old? What it was like to be called to dinner when you were outside having the time of your life playing tag with your friends? To be made to come in, to sit down, to sit still, to finish your meal? I was the youngest of four and my mother had the toughest time getting us all to sit in one spot to eat. There was always so much going on that I remember sitting at the table like I had ants in my pants.

In fact, my mom used to constantly ask me if I actually did, have ants in my pants. I just couldn't sit still. I was the type of kid who would run to the table, take a bite of food and then run around the house eight or nine times before I settled back in for another bite. As a result, I rarely finished a meal and it drove my mother crazy.

But here's the thing, when I was five or six years old, I had the most adorable little set of abs that you've ever seen. I was ripped. I'm talking, zero cellulite. I looked amazing. Maybe I was on to something. Maybe sitting at a table with a big plate of food, my feet up, watching television, isn't the best way to eat a meal. Maybe

I should run to the table, grab a bite of food and then run around the house. Maybe we all should go back to acting like a bunch of kids.

"A game of tag anyone?"

**Be the type of person who would rather act like a kid, running around the house like you have ants in your pants, than the grown adult who barely moves and finishes everything that is on their plate... because of the, you know... starving children in Africa and all.

36. KEEP FOOD OUT OF REACH

I grew up in a large family, six of us, plus a cousin or two, plus the neighbor kids, and my mom would always make a lot of food and put it all on the table. Then we'd eat, and visit, and eat some more, and continue to visit. Some of us would smoke. All of us would continue to pick at the food, even though we had finished eating 30 minutes earlier.

I carried this practice into my adulthood. I would make a bunch of food, (okay, so I would order a bunch of food) and bring it all to the table with me. It didn't matter if I was eating alone, or with family and friends; all the food would go onto the table and we would eat, and visit, and eat some more.

I had to break that habit. Now, whether I'm cooking for myself or ordering in, I make my plate up in the kitchen, careful to put only what I am going to eat. Everything else gets left behind and put away when I'm done.

**Be the type of person that keeps food out of reach. The type of person who knows the dangers of sitting next to a big basket of bread, or a pan full of lasagna and doesn't put themselves in that situation.

37. KICK YOUR OWN ASS

As much as I waited and waited for someone or something to get me off the couch, to help me from eating eight times a day, or to make better food choices for me, and to actually get me to go to the gym, it never happened. No one ever came to my rescue. No one ever took the fork away from me, or rolled me out of bed in the morning and made me go to the gym or turned off my television. In the end, I had to kick my own ass.

The truth is, it doesn't matter how many diet books you buy or what gym you belong too or how new and form fitting your running shoes are. It doesn't matter what diet plan you follow or what the scale says or how many times you dream of being thinner, healthier, and sexier. Until you get up and start kicking your own ass, none of it is ever going to matter. None of it, is ever going to work.

I cannot tell you how many times I have screamed at myself in the mirror. Literally, hating myself for not staying on track, for not following my diet, for the way I looked and felt. I deserved better and I knew it. But for some reason, I was always looking for and hoping, someone or something would come along and make me do it. That's all I needed, I thought. Someone else.

Then April 25th happened and I woke up fat... I won't bore you with the details (again), other than to say that the one of the things that separated April 24th from April 25 was the realization that it was all on me. No one was coming to my rescue. If I truly wanted to shut up that little whiney voice in my head, I had to do it myself. I had to start kicking my own ass.

**I hope you are the type of person who doesn't have to hit rock bottom and then fall down a set of concrete steps into a pool, in order to take control, and start kicking your own ass. Be the type of person who kicks your own ass.

38. GET OFF THE SCALE

I know, I know... Make up my mind. First I tell you to get on the scale and now I'm telling you to get off the scale. What's the answer?

The truth is, both. The best thing about scales is they tell you how much progress you've made. The worst thing about scales, if used inappropriately, is they give you an excuse to eat a little of this, and a little of that... and that will make you fat.

It's called the "Scale Game," and it goes like this.

You finally get over your fear of the scale and you start weighing yourself every day. Big mistake.

If you are like me, if you weigh yourself every day, you start making "food" decisions based on what the scale says that morning. If I was down a half pound between yesterday and today (and that happens; your weight fluctuates throughout the week, the day, the hour and so on...) I would use that small success to justify the second helping, the small piece of cake, the ice cream, whatever... And then, of course, I would weigh myself on Saturday morning, the ONLY morning I was supposed to weigh myself, and guess what... I would be up.

**Be the type of person who doesn't play the scale game. The type of person who picks one day a week (at the same time of day) to weigh themselves and then puts the scale away, until the following week.

39. DEVELOP A MORNING ROUTINE

I read a great book called <u>The Miracle Morning</u> by Hal Elrod (2015) that completely transformed my mornings and hence, my life.

In his book, Hal tries to persuade you to stop lollygagging in bed, with little to no agenda, or mission or routine to follow. I went from a diehard believer of needing eight hours of sleep a night, and waking up with little or no routine (except for the bathroom, teeth, coffee routine), to figuring out that I really only needed six hours of sleep at night, and designing a morning routine that has enabled me to get a jump start on my reading, my writing, self-discovery and exercise. All of which, are very important to me. As a frame of reference, here is my typical morning routine.

- Bed by 10pmWake up at 4am
- Do 100 pushups, or as many as I can

- Drink 16 oz of water – from beside my bed (at room temperature: see Cameron Diaz's book "The Body Book" (2013))
- Grab a book (chosen the night before) and set the timer on my phone for 30 minutes
- Meditate: Set alarm for 10 minutes and find a comfortable spot and try to clear my head
- Get coffee
- Free Write: Set my alarm for 10 minutes and type as fast as I can – with my eyes closed
- Write: Set my alarm for 30 minutes and write meaningfully
- 6am: Exercise (I follow a set schedule / routine)
- 7 – 8am:
  - ◊ Shower
  - ◊ Eat Breakfast

I follow this routine seven days a week and it has proven to be extremely helpful. Keep in mind, losing weight is not about losing weight. It is about changing your life. It is about living with intention. It is about setting yourself up for success. What better way to ensure that you are going to be successful, than to start each morning with the knowledge and intention of doing things that make you happy.

**Be the type of person who no longer lays around in bed, waiting until you feel like getting up, or worse, absolutely have too. The type of person who no longer lets life come to them, but rather the type of person that goes out and gets what they want and need, intentionally.

40. PRE-TRACK

I'll be honest, I am an excellent tracker when it comes to breakfast and lunch. Dinner... However, not so much. I'd love to tell you it is because I am so super busy in the evening, and that I just don't think of it, but I'd be lying. Here's the truth.

Dinner is always on the fence with me. It doesn't matter what I 'planned' to eat, as much as it matters who's around and what I'm doing and what I feel like having to eat. Then, another truth, if I don't track, it is because tracking was either too hard, or I just don't want to know how many points I just ate.

Pre-tracking is made up of two parts. It is one part 'proactively tracking' and one part sticking to your plan.

If you are planning your meals in advance, measuring everything out and know what you are going to eat and when, then take a few minutes in the morning and pre-track all of the food you are planning on eating. If you deviate from any of this, just make the adjustment.

**Be the type of person who keeps track of what you eat, or pre-tracks.

41. CHEAT ON LUNCH, NOT YOURSELF

I would start at McDonald's for breakfast. Then move on to Wendy's or Burger King for lunch and then order take-out pizza and wings or worse, Chinese food for dinner. I did this every Sunday when I was dieting. It was my cheat day.

For years and years, I struggled with my weight and for years and years, every time I started a diet I would include a "cheat day." And cheat, I did. I ate like an idiot from the time I got up to the time I went to bed.

The problem with a "cheat day" is it would cancel out all of the hard work I did all week. It didn't matter how well I did, or how many times I was able to put my fork down, or not go up for seconds, as soon as Sunday came, I would eat and eat and eat. Eventually, I realized that I was cheating myself.

**Be the type of person who has a cheat meal, instead of a whole day. Be the type of person that begins and ends every day, with a healthy meal. Be the type of person who cheats on lunch, not themselves.

42. STOP TRYING TO EAT HEALTHY

"I'm trying to be good," I say. Or, "I'm trying to eat healthy," I lie. The truth is, every time I have used that statement, in response to someone asking me if I wanted to go somewhere to get some food, I am testing the waters. I am looking for some commiseration.

I want the person that I am talking to, to shake their head and give me the same sentiment in response. "Me too," I want them to say. "I too, am trying to be good. To eat healthy."

By doing this, we are both acknowledging how tough it is to "be good," or "eat healthy," and therefore, giving each other a pass.

Permission to eat like an asshole. It is as if we both just agreed that life is too short, eating healthy is too hard, and you know... "We are all going to die of something..."

Stop "trying" to eat healthy and just do it. Stop buying food that you shouldn't have, or going to places you shouldn't be, or hanging out with people who are just "trying" to eat healthy. Toughen up. Kick your own ass (Rule #37).

**Be the type of person who is a healthy eater. Period. No more excuses. No more, "I'm trying." Be the type of person who just "is" a healthy eater.

43. IT DOESN'T MATTER WHEN YOU ARE DONE

I had one of those profound "A-ha" moments a couple of years ago, that I hope I am able to articulate. Here we go:

> *It doesn't matter what I ate, when I was done eating.*

Let me explain.

It was one of those (thousands) of times that I was in a grocery store looking for something healthy to eat for lunch, while craving everything that was unhealthy. It was the kind of grocery store that has a large food court in it. One were you can get pizza and sushi, and panini's and coffee and donuts. The kind that has eight differ-ent buffet tables with everything from soup and salad to Chinese food to chicken wings and "Specialty Chef" creations. Those places are tough to shop in when your fat and struggling.

There I was, walking though the food court and coming up with every excuse in the world on why I could... no... should... maybe even deserved, an egg roll with a side of General Tso Chicken, pork fried rice and some dumplings. Maybe even a couple of chicken wings – oh, and a few cheese sticks.

Of course, five minutes later I give in and get the stupid Chinese food and chicken wings and, because I'm the dumbest person on the planet, grab a large chocolate chip cookie that is on display at the register. (Isn't it funny how, if you let yourself cheat a little, you go overboard, and cheat a lot? Is it just me?)

Five minutes later I'm sitting in my car stuffing my face. I'm not driving. The food smells amazing and I can't believe that I gave in and let myself have such a wonderful treat. I'm using both hands, shoveling it in as fast as I can. It's as if I am scared that I could change my mind at any moment and throw it all away. I don't want to throw it away.

Another ten minutes and I'm on the road, I find a radio station and settle in for another hour or so of driving. That's when it hits me. The full feeling. I look over at the carnage in the passenger seat. The tore open packages, the plastic containers, and the used napkins. I'm no longer hungry. Then, the "A-ha" moment.

I could have eaten anything just now. I could have had grilled chicken and cherry tomatoes or a cup of chicken noodle soup with a small bag of oyster crackers, or humus with carrot sticks. I could have eaten anything and felt the same way that I did right then. Full. No longer hungry. No longer craving anything. Satisfied.

It turns out, it doesn't matter what you eat, when you are done eating. You can't taste and enjoy a slice of pizza ten minutes after you eat it. A bowl of ice cream, when it's gone, no longer tastes good... so why not eat healthy?

**Be the type of person who understands that it is not going to matter what you ate, after you are done eating it. The type of person who eats plain chicken and raw vegetables, instead of beer battered chicken wings and fried rice – because you now... it is not going to matter, when you are done.

44. EARN A MEDAL

There has been a huge debate going on for a while now, regarding participation medals, awards and the increasingly popular, mini graduations. I'll admit it, I agreed with the masses that said giving everyone a participation medal or an award just for being there, or having every grade from kindergarten through junior high have its own graduation, was foolish at best, and could be damaging at worst.

"What are we teaching our kids," I would have said. "If everyone gets an award, doesn't that lessen the very idea of an award?"

Up to this point I had never won anything. Not in my whole life; I have never come in first or second or even third... in any-thing. I have never won a trophy, a certificate, a ribbon or a medal. In fact, most of the time, I was the last kid picked. Then I earned my first medal and everything changed.

You know the story. I woke up fat... Yada yada yada... I started walking. After a while, I began jogging between telephone poles until I could run. Then I started running. Slow at first and not very far, but I was running.

After a few months, I started entering 5k races and mud races and color races and it was a lot of fun. I got a few cool T shirts, but no medal. Medals were only for the top three athletes. Something I knew, I would never be. Then my friend asked if I wanted to run a half marathon with him. A half marathon... as in, 13.1 miles. I didn't think I could, but he assured me. "All we have to do is train," he said. And we did.

A few months later, with one of my best friends in the whole world Eric, we laced up our shoes and ran the farthest distance either of us had ever run. I remember getting to the finish line, completely exhausted, overwhelmed with emotion and in a lot of pain. Then they presented me with a finishers medal and that was it. I couldn't hold back the tears. I did it. I ran 13.1 miles and I had proof.

Finisher medals are just that. Proof of participation. I walked around with that medal for days. I wore it at the airport. I wore it to work, and even pulled it out at the dentist to show everyone. I could not have been more proud of that medal. Of me. And, I couldn't wait to earn another one.

**Be the type of person who goes out and pushes themselves beyond what they think is possible. The type of person who goes so far, and works so hard, that they earn a medal. I hope it turns you into the type of person who wants to earn more.

45. STOP TELLING EVERYONE YOU'RE DIETING

This is a real challenge. Telling someone that you are dieting is making an excuse for your healthy eating habits. It's as if you are admitting that you are punishing yourself for bad behavior.

The truth is, you need to stop eating shit food, because shit food is no good. You are not dieting, you are a healthy eater. Say it out loud. "I am a healthy eater."

Come on... say out loud. "I am a healthy eater."

Change your response to people who question what you are eating to a proud statement of, "I don't eat that kind of stuff" instead of, "That is not on my diet. I'm being punished."

That is not on my diet, is a turn of phrase that says, I can and will eat it at some other time, a time when I am not feeling so bad about myself.

But here is the thing, you feel bad about yourself because of those shit foods. There will never be a time when eating shitty food leads to good feelings. Ever.

**Be the type of person who stops dieting and starts living a healthy life style. The type of person who has a list of foods that they simply do not eat because they are not good for you.

46. STUFF YOUR WEIGHT IN A SACK

It had been a few weeks of eating right, moving more, and keeping strict track of everything I was eating, and I still wasn't losing any weight. I was down about thirty pounds, but had plateaued. I had fallen into a slump and I was miserable.

Then I caught an episode of the television show, The Biggest Loser – which is a reality tv show about weight loss. In the episode, I watched, each contestant had to put all the weight they had lost, up to that point (for some it was over 100lbs), into a bag and drag it across a football field. It was amazing.

I remember running down stairs, to where I kept all of my unused gym equipment, and grabbed 30lbs of weights and put them into a back pack. Holy moly, that thing was heavy. I couldn't believe I had lost that much weight. I brought the bag upstairs and for weeks I picked it up, or put the back pack on and marveled at how heavy it was. Any time anyone came over I would tell them to pick it up. Everyone was amazed and impressed.

I love this tip. Maybe you've had some success in the beginning, but now find yourself in a slump. Maybe it's been a few weeks since you've lost weight. Maybe your frustrated and want to throw in the towel. Maybe you don't realize just how much weight you have really lost. If so, this tip is for you. Find some weights, or rocks, or gallons of water, whatever equals the amount of weight you've lost and stuff all the weight into a sack and then pick it up. Repeat as needed.

**Be the type of person who keeps things in perspective. The type of person who stuffs their weight into a sack and then carries it around like a trophy; because it is... and you should be proud of yourself.

47. SPIT IT OUT

I remember watching the Rocky Marciano story years ago, (it's about a boxer who is having a less than mediocre career until he decides to go Pro). Like all movies do, there is a montage of scenes that shows all the various stages of training that he goes through (usually to some uplifting theme music).

During the montage, there is this reoccurring scene where Rocky is having dinner with his parents. His mother, just learning of his new diet restrictions is beside herself. He won't eat bread, or tomatoes, and when it comes to steak... he spits it out.

"I can't swallow the steak, I can only swallow the juice."

"You can't swallow the steak?"

"I got to lose weight Ma."

"We finally get steak in the house and he can't eat it..."

. . . .

I will admit that I do this mostly with donuts. I don't know why I have such a craving sometimes for donuts, but I do. I just love them. That is, I love the taste of them. I don't love how it makes me feel or look. So sometimes, when I am having a craving for a donut, I have a donut, but I don't eat it.

I take a bite, chew it. It's delicious. I spit it out.

** Be the type of person who goes Pro in their weight loss efforts. Buy, bite, chew, savor the goodness, but then spit it out.

48. EMBRACE THE COLD

Michael Phelps is the most decorated Olympian in history, with a grand total of 23 Olympic titles and 28 medals. In 2008, during the Beijing Olympics, he set the world on fire with his unbelievably fast swimming abilities. Soon everyone wanted to know everything about him. They wanted to know what time he woke up in the morning; what time he went to bed, how long he trained for, how long he spent in the pool, and of course, what his diet consisted of.

I remember watching everything about him. The swimming, the training, the random shots of him with his swim team and all the interviews.

"Eat, sleep, swim," he said. That's all he does. "4,000 calories per meal," he said. Four-thousand calories per meal! That's a staggering 12,000 calories a day. It didn't take long before one expert after another to begin analyzing his caloric intake claim. No one believed him.

It's hard to imagine how anyone could swim enough to burn 12,000 calories a day, they reasoned. It's impossible, some said. But then, someone analyzed the water temperature. On average, Michael Phelps was swimming (at an Olympic pace) between two and three hours a day in a pool that was 68° Fahrenheit.

Meaning, in addition to swimming for hours, at a very fast pace, his body had to work extra hard to keep warm. "Hmm...," I thought. "I should go out in the cold more often."

**Be the type of person who embraces the cold. The type of person that ditches the heavy jacket for a lighter one. The type of person who is willing to shiver.

49. DON'T GO HUNGRY

"I don't understand," I said. I was at a cocktail party and saw a guy looking at all the hors d'oeuvres, but not eating any. I told him that I felt his pain. All the hors d'oeuvres were either fried or battered, and none of them were healthy.

"Yeah, I go hungry a lot," he said smiling.

"You go hungry," I repeated, not sure if he was telling me the truth.

"I'm a vegan," he said. "And if you're truly committed to being a vegan, like I am, then you go hungry sometimes," he shrugged. "It's just the way it is."

"A vegan," I said nodding. "How about that." He laughed.

Recently, for a reason I can't really explain, I decided that I wanted to try fasting. You know, the kind where you go without food for a few days, or a few weeks. I decided that I was going to go five days without food. The only thing I would have was water and black coffee. That's it.

The first two days were not terrible. It was a bit tough, but hunger doesn't escalate, meaning, hunger pains go away after a few minutes. This was a great revelation. However, when I woke up on the third day, I was fit to be tied. I couldn't concentrate. I couldn't stop thinking about food and I my stomach was killing me. I felt bloated and nauseous.

By 3pm, I had enough and went on a tear. I had a protein shake, and then I went to a burger joint right around the corner from my house, and had a cheese burger and fries – something that I hadn't had in a long time. On my way home I stopped at a frozen yogurt place and filled one of those large containers with every topping they had, coconut ice cream and caramel sauce. By the time I got home it was 4:30 in the afternoon. By 7pm, I was hungry again and went out for a couple of slices of pizza.

The whole time I was gorging myself, I was thinking that I had gone without food for two and a half days, so none of this really mattered. Heck, I deserved it.

I gained weight that week. And that guy, in the beginning, the Vegan, although he claimed to go hungry for his cause sometimes, he too was overweight – by a lot. That is why you should never go hungry.

For me, skipping a couple of meals, makes me think I can splurge on the next couple. I can't. It doesn't work that way. It is best to be prepared and eat when you are supposed to eat.

**Be the type of person who doesn't go hungry. The type of person who doesn't give themselves any excuse to overeat. The type of person who is always prepared and always eats when they are supposed to.

50. STOP ACTING LIKE A COW

I have tried so many different diets and weight loss challenges and read so many books and considered so many different opinions that sometimes, I feel like I am too smart for my own good. All the advice seems to blend together and I'm not sure if I am coming or going. Am I supposed to be eating three times a day or six? Should I schedule my meals or wait until I'm hungry before I eat? What if I'm only sort of hungry, but not really? Should I snack or wait it out? What should I be snacking on?

Before long, my attempts at trying to figure what I'm supposed to do, and not being completely committed to one idea or another, I would end up spending my days grazing like a big fat cow. And, like a cow, I continually gained weight. Aimlessly eating all day, i.e. grazing, regardless of the food I was grazing on, always led to overeating. And overeating always led to gaining weight. I had to stop acting like a cow.

If you are hungry enough to eat, then eat a full meal. Not a part of a meal, or a few bites of this or that throughout the day; eat a full meal. Meals should be specific, measured, and timed. They should be an event all on their own. If you really want to lose weight, you should stop acting like a cow. Stop grazing.

**Be the type of person who doesn't spend all day eating. The type of person who doesn't leave food out so every time you walk by you are tempted to reach, to taste, to nibble and graze. Be the type of person who doesn't want to be the size of a cow. The type that doesn't act like one.

CHAPTER EIGHT

Losing weight is not about losing weight.

"Lose Weight Now, Ask Me How," her button said. We were at the Sky View Casino, a local dance spot that had live music every Friday and Saturday night and drew families (like mine) in from all over the area, who were looking for something to do.

"How," I said pointing to her button. She looked at me from head to toe. I was fifteen years old, tall, lanky, and I didn't have a stitch of body fat. She smiled.

"You don't need to lose any weight," she said dismissing me.

"No," I said. "But my mom and dad does." She laughed out loud, recognizing I was a bit of smart ass. "I'm serious," I said. "They're huge."

"Well," she said. "Are your parents here?" I nodded and pointed to the back corner of the room where my mom and dad were snacking on popcorn and Doritos, drinking booze and having a great time. She looked at them, and then back at me. A guy (her husband maybe), stood up from the table and gave me a business card. It said "Herbalife" on it.

"Give this to your parents and tell them that if they are serious about losing weight, to come on over here and talk to us," he said. I smiled, telling them I would. Then I ran back to my parents table and announced that I had finally found the cure for them being so fat.

See, I didn't just wake up fat. I grew up fat. My parents struggled with their weight my whole life, and probably most of their own. I feel like I have spent my whole childhood watching Guiding Light, and listening to my parents talk about (and try) every diet program they could find. My mom was a huge fan of bringing home grocery store tablets; those pocket-sized magazines you find at the cash register, each touting the latest diet craze. There was Dexatrim (the diet pill), and Slim Fast, (a shake that came in metal cans and tasted like chalk). Then there was the Oat Bran diet and the Grape Fruit diet and aerobics with Jane Fonda and, of course, the Richard

Simons Show. My parents even had this fat jiggling machine, (a Vibrating Belt Machine) that they would get on in an attempt to break up the body fat to lose weight. As if the fat was simply stuck inside of them and all it needed was a good jiggling to come loose.

I can't begin to tell you how funny it was every time my mom or dad got on that thing, or how many times my brothers, sister and I got in trouble for trying to play on it. Eventually though, the Vibrating Belt Machine, (like all exercise equipment I came to learn) lost its appeal and was pushed into the corner of the living room where it began its new career as a coat rack.

But I didn't just grow up fat. Like growing up Catholic or Jewish, I grew up a smoker and a drinker and an overeater. I grew up learning how to act by watching, believing and eventually emulating everything my parents did. My parents overate, so I grew up overeating. My parents were smokers, so I grew up a smoker. My dad was a heavy drinker and a curser, and so I too would become a heavy drinker and I still curse.

More than just emulating action, however, I grew up with the same outlook and attitude toward life as my parents had. I remember learning about the dangers of cigarettes smoking in the fourth or fifth grade and coming home and telling my dad about it. About how my teacher told us that cigarettes were bad for you and that they caused cancer and you could die if you smoked them.

"We are all going to die of something," my dad said. We were at the dinner table still eating when my dad lit up. It wasn't just a throw away statement, either, it was truly how he viewed life. As if not being able to stop death was an excuse for not having to take responsibility for anything. More than just my dad, however, my parents, my aunts and uncles and indeed, everyone I was exposed to, had this victim mentality. Nothing was ever their fault. Everything was always happening to them. And, like the eventuality of death, there was no use in fighting it.

In fact, my parents always struggled. Always tried to live off whatever was given to them, whether it was a meaningless job for little or no money, or if it was government assistance. I don't mean to say that they didn't try or that they didn't want more out of life, they did, but... "We are all going to die of something..."

I remember the day that changed my life like it was yesterday. There were a couple of times. A few notable instances that I should tell you about, but the first one happened when I was 22 years old. I was a high school dropout ("because we are all going to die of something..."), working in a job I hated and for a boss that I hated even more. I worked in construction as a laborer.

It was the middle of December and I had just gotten laid off, like I always did in the winter. I had heard that there was another construction site, about an hour and fifteen minutes away from my house that wasn't shutting down for the winter (like most had).

I had this piece of crap Ford Escort that could barely get out of its own way, but decided to drive the distance to see if I could get some work. The foreman was a real asshole who just took down my number, saying he would call if anything came up, but he was sure nothing would. Angry and depressed, I left.

There were two ways I could go to get back to my place. The way that I came, which took about an hour and fifteen minutes, or a shorter way, up and over Lincoln Gap. They closed the Gap down at some point in the winter, because it would eventually become too hazardous to travel on, but for now it was still open. I should have given it more thought as to whether my car could make it over the Gap or not, but having just wasted my entire morning, not to mention all the gas I had, just to get turned away at the job site pissed me off. "F' it," I thought and just went for it.

The mountain however, proved to be too steep for my crappy car and just before I made it to the top of the Gap, smoke started to pour from the engine; it spat and sputtered for a few more yards and then overheated. I put my foot on the brake, so I didn't roll back down the hill, and sat there. I sat there, staring out the window, at all the smoke, my hands gripping the steering wheel so tight that my forearms began to burn. Then came the tears. I was so frustrated and mad.

I put the car in park, stepped on the emergency brake and then, as if the steering wheel was the reason for all my problems, I began pounding on it and screaming and crying. I couldn't believe this was my life. I hated working in construction. I hated my car, my apartment, my girlfriend, my lot in life, my boss, that stupid asshole foreman, always getting laid off, struggling from one paycheck to another, my upbringing, my parents... but most of all, I hated myself.

I got out of the car, slamming the door harder than I should have, and lit a cigarette ("because we are all going to die of something..."). Then it began to snow. I remember laughing through gritted teeth. Of course, it was snowing. I opened the hood and knew that I just had to wait for the car to cool down and then it would start again. I got back in the car, turned the key on and searched the radio dial.

"...If you don't like where you are in your life, then move. If you don't like your career, or you don't know anything else, then go back to school and learn something. Get a new skill, a new job... heck, a new career.

You live in the greatest country in the world. You can do and have and be anything and everything you want..."

I had no idea who was talking on the radio and would later learn that the guy's name was Rush Limbaugh. I had never heard of him before. I had never heard anyone talk like him. And although he wasn't talking to me, he may as well have been. The guy on the phone started pushing back, making excuses. Just like I would have.

"Stop," Rush said. "Stop blaming everyone else. The only thing stopping you, is you." Then he paused for a moment, collecting his thoughts. I leaned in, desperate to hear more.

"This is a real problem folks. I hope you are listening to this guy. We are afforded more opportunities in this country, than any other country in the world, but it doesn't just come to you. You have to go out there and work for it." (I am paraphrasing).

It didn't happen right away. It wasn't as if my car started right up and I drove up and over the hill and into the most perfect life imaginable – just because I heard some guy on the radio yell at another guy on the radio for acting like a victim. But it changed my perspective. He changed the way I viewed myself, my upbringing and more importantly, my future. Rush Limbaugh saved my life.

From then on, I vowed to be in control. To be accountable and responsible for everything that did and did not happen to me. I drove up and over that mountain that day, still broke, still unemployed, still hating my lot in life... but I drove up and over that mountain with a different attitude. My eyes were open. I was not going to be a victim anymore. I didn't like where I was, or what I was doing or who I was with or the amount of money that I earned, and I know knew, that if I wanted it to change, then I was going to have to change it. I didn't have to settle for what everyone else thought I was worth. I lived in the greatest country in the world. I'm an American. And there is this dream. Maybe you've heard of it. The American Dream. And now, I was going to find it and live it.

Fast forward 8 years, and I am just about to graduate with my first Bachelor's degree (That's right! A bachelor's degree! I went from a high school drop out to a college graduate, not once, but four times... that is, (at the time of this writing anyway, I have four college degrees!). I'm telling you... Rush Limbaugh saved my life. But I digress.

I came across a book by Glenn Beck called "The Real America: Messages from the Heart and Heartland," (2010). In that book, Glenn points out that most of us, when we talk to our children about their future, (and indeed, whenever anyone talked to us about ours when we were kids), always asked "what" we wanted to be when we grew up. Which drew responses like, "I want to be a Police Officer," or "I want to be a Doctor."

The problem with this kind of questioning, Glenn says. Is it misses the mark. The most valuable question we should be asking our kids, and most importantly, to ourselves is, "Who" do we want to be?

That is, what kind of a person are you going to be? What kind of person do you want to be? Do you want to be the type of person that sticks up for others, or are you going to be the type of person that looks the other way, or worse, one that takes advantage? Do you want to be the type of person that says please and thank you, or the type the just expects people to do things for you? Do you want to be the type of person that stays until their work is finished or the type that leaves everything half done?

What kind of parent do you want to be? What kind of daughter or son, or neighbor, community member, manager, employee, friend, husband, or wife? Who do you want to be?

The questions are endless, but they all reinforce the most valuable lesson that Rush Limbaugh was speaking about 8 years earlier. It is all up to me. I get to decide what kind of person I am going to be. Am I going to be the type of person who, like I was raised, never puts the grocery cart back where I got it from, instead, just pushing it between cars, or rolling it away, not caring where it goes? (I'm providing job security for someone... I would mimic, after hearing it said hundreds of times). Am I going to be the type that grabs and eats grapes on the way into a supermarket? Or the type that throws trash on the ground without any thought to who is going to pick it up? Or the type of person who spends all the money they ever made? Am I going to be the type of person who smokes and drinks and over eats because... "I'm going to die of something anyway..." Or am I going to be different.

One of my favorite sayings on this subjects is from the late Zig Ziglar. He says, "If you don't like were you are right now, leave. You are not a tree!" It makes me laugh every time I think about it. I'm not a tree, and I'm going to go out on a limb here and say, if you are reading this, then there is a good chance that you too, are not a tree.

In the end, if you are serious about losing weight, then you need to change your life. That is what I've learned through this entire process. I needed to change the way that I saw myself. How I treated myself. How I let others treat me. It is about deciding to live with intention. Deciding once and for all, what kind of person you are going to be... and then taking the steps to become that person.

Be the type of person who pees in the woods....
Be the type of person who stays off the grass....
Be the type of person who burns their fat clothes....
Be the type of person who keeps track of everything they eat....
Be the type of person who gets new friends...
Be the type of person who puts themselves first...

CHAPTER NINE

Run For Your Life

The race consisted of six laps around a four-mile loop. It was February, in Grand Rapids Michigan and the path was snow covered except for a one mile stretch between the second and third mile. My rubber studded cleats made their final click, clack sound as I left the bare pavement for the last time.

There were two Aid stations placed at mile one and three, and each time I passed, the volunteers would shake noisy cowbells and clap and smile and offer water, Gatorade, Mountain Dew and cookies. It was 8° when we started, and by the time I was on my last lap (four hours later) the temperature had risen to 12°.

All the volunteers had been out there the whole time, in a constant state of motion, trying to stay warm and cheery for the runners.

"Hey guys," I said, taking off my face mask and gloves so that I could talk and fist bump all of them.

"I can't thank you guys enough for being out here;" I said. "Braving this cold weather to support all of the runners." I extended my fist. "I really appreciate it."

A couple of runners had caught up to me when I was speaking. "We," I said gesturing to them. Everyone laughed. "We all appreciate you guys for being out here." They smiled and nodded in agreement as they grabbed some water and continued to run.

"This is my first marathon," someone announced from behind me. I turned around and saw this young guy hunched over. He had his hands on his knees, straining to look up at me. Exhausted.

"Is that true," I said. He nodded and smiled. Then he let his head hang, stretching out the back of his neck.

"That's awesome," I said. "You've got to let me run the last couple of miles with you."

"That'd be great," he said. "This is a lot harder than I thought it would be."

"I know," I said and we left.

He told me his name was Jeromy, he was 27 years old, and for the life of him, he couldn't quite explain why he decided to run a marathon.

"I've been thinking about running a marathon for a long time," he said. "At least try. To see if I could do it. To push myself."

"So great," I said and started to well up with emotion. I don't know what it is, but I get super emotional at the end of a marathon. It's embarrassing really. Most people are hooting and hollering when they cross the finish line and there I am, barely holding it together.

The night before my first marathon my friend Jessica sent me an encouraging text.

"Ralph, I'm thinking of you. I'm so proud of you and how far you have come. Run will all of your strength tomorrow, until your whole body wants to quit, then run with heart."

I think about that text every time I'm at the end of a race and my body starts to break down. "Run with heart," I say to myself. "Don't give up. Don't stop. Go... Go... Go..." By the time I get to the finish line, I am exhausted and emotionally spent.

Now, running with this guy, who is the same age as my son, my emotions get the best of me and for a few minutes we just run. I have this urge to tell him all about myself. About waking up fat, and drunk and hating myself and I want to warn him. Instead, I told him about Mr. Reynold's.

. . . .

"Why are you so fat," he said when I sat down beside him. I laughed.

"Mr. Reynold's!" a nurse said, giving him a look. I waved her off.

"No worries," I said. I work in long term care and the elderly I've learned, don't have much of a filter.

"Guess how old I am," he said sitting up taller. I looked at him, not sure if I should guess high or low.

"Eighty," I said.

"N.i.n.e.t.y – t.w.o." he said stretching the word out. I whistled. "Do you know what the worst thing about getting old is?" I didn't.

"Everyone I know is dead." I looked at him. "Everyone," he said. "Dead!" He smiled, though not in a funny way and shook his head. "All my friends, my siblings, everyone I grew up with. Even my younger brother, who was five years younger than me. Dead!" I looked over at the nurse to see if she was still listening but she wasn't. I didn't know what to do or say, so I just sat there.

After a couple of minutes Mr. Reynold's leaned over.

"Want to know how I did it," he said. He had big bushy white eyebrows and he raised one at me. I nodded and leaned in closer.

"I started running when I turned fifty."

"Running," I said.

"I was just like you," he said sitting back in his chair. "Not as fat, but out of shape. I smoked cigarettes and drank booze and spent more time sitting on my ass than I should have. Then I turned fifty... the big 5.0. and that was it. I quit all of it and started running."

"Running," I said again. He nodded slowly, thinking, remembering. "I wish I could run," I said.

"I have run a marathon in every state, on every continent, in some of the worst conditions and some of the best. I've seen the entire world on my feet." He smiled.

"That's the way you do it," he said, leaning in again. "That's how you outlive everyone. Not like that!" He shook his head in disgust, while staring at my stomach.

. . . .

"How many marathons have you run," Jeromy asked.

"This is my 29th marathon, and 24th state."

"Are you going to run in every state?"

"Every state and every continent," I said, then we heard the cheers. We were on the home stretch, a half mile to go.

"When we get to the end of that fence," I said pointing. "We have to pick up our pace so we look good when we finish." Jeromy laughed but nodded.

As we passed the fence and began to pick up the pace, I wished I had the opportunity to see Mr. Reynold's again. To thank him for telling me his story. To show him.

About a hundred yards from the finish line Jeromy started to fall back a bit, so I slowed down. I didn't want to beat him. I wanted to finish with him.

"Stay strong," I said. We entered the cattle shoot together and

I raised my hands in the air, trying to get the crowd to cheer. They did.

I turned around after getting my medal and looked for Jeromy. He was being swallowed up in a huge bear hug from his parents. I waited. When they let go, he saw me.

"Thank you," he said extending his hand. I took it and we shook and half hugged. "I don't know if I could have finished without you." I smiled, knowing the feeling.

"Dad. This guy has run 29 marathons."

"Wow," his dad said.

"I'm Ralph," I said shaking his hand. Then I turned back to Jeromy and grabbed him by the shoulder.

"Keep running," I said. "Make it part of your life. Run for your life. It's worth it. You are worth it." He smiled and hugged me again.

"I will," he said. "I really will."

CHAPTER 10

Why me... Why this Story

*"Someday we'll look back on this
and it will all seem funny. Fa La La..."*

-BRUCE SPRINGSTEEN (ROSALITA)

Hello everyone, I'm Ralph Peterson and I used to weigh 350lbs... The story you just read is true. Waking up fat, hitting rock bottom and then falling down the stairs... the timing... a clear view... needing a witness, being scared shitless, the adventures in Dietland, and learning the very important lesson, that losing weight is not about losing weight, really happened.

However, as hard as all of that was to go through, deciding to share my story, continues to be one of the hardest.

I'm embarrassed. I don't know how else to say it. While I am extremely proud of myself for being able to take control of my life; to quit drinking, to go back to school, to work hard, and to lose the weight, the irony of it all is not lost on me; I wasn't supposed to abuse alcohol, or smoke cigarettes or eat so much that I nearly killed myself. I am not blameless. And in that sense, I sometimes feel like a fraud.

"You should have met Ralph a few years ago," I overhear one of my friends say to someone we are just meeting. They are proud of me and can't help but share my story, to brag. For me, it feels like I am getting sucker punched. My face gets red hot with embarrassment and I want to crawl under the nearest rock.

Then that person tells another person, who tells someone else, and that person contacts me and asks to hear my story. She is looking for guidance, for help... for proof that it's possible.

I remember calling her and still not being sure if I wanted to tell my story. I was still embarrassed. But then she told me hers. She told me how depressed and angry she was. 'The heaviest she's ever been,' she said. Her desperation was palatable. I've been there... so I started talking.

Once I started, of course, I couldn't stop. We talked for hours and I told her everything. I told her about the Bahamas and wanting to throw myself off the balcony. About the hopeless feeling and the anger. I told her all of it. Sometimes we laughed; sometimes we cried. She said she was writing down everything I was saying. I couldn't believe it. I was helping. My story was making a difference!

We both hung up the phone different people that day. She was more determined than ever to get her life back and I had found my voice – my purpose.

I'm Ralph Peterson, and I used to weigh 350lbs and I am living proof that if I can do it... Then you can do it.

It is going to take work. It's not going to be easy. It is going to require some planning and some changes and deciding to live your life with intention, but it is worth it. You are worth it.

Cheers!

Ralph

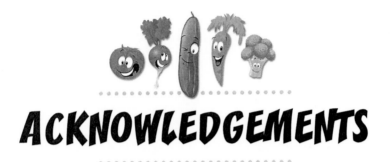

ACKNOWLEDGEMENTS

Anytime anyone goes through a life changing event, as I have, it is hard to pinpoint every single person who checked in with me, gave me guidance, offered me their ear, their couches, their love, support and sometimes even a couple of bucks. To all of you – everyone who has ever helped, or even offered to help me get through this, I am forever grateful.

There are a handful of people that need special recognition for going way above and beyond; ensuring that I was staying on track and always moving in the right direction.

Most notably, my best friends and go to confidants: Adam Duke, Devan Luciano, Eric Preus, Sandy Sarza, Lori Shibinette and Kerry Winger.

Adam Duke, who is the most persistent (some may say nagging) man I have ever known. He is singlehandedly responsible for me sitting down and writing this book. "Is it done yet?" Devan Luciano, who has spent years and years listening, arguing, supporting and vetting every decision I've ever made. Eric Preus. I'm not sure where to begin. Perhaps when we were 12 or 13 years old, running on the back side of the river, kicking a can back and forth and dreaming of one day running a marathon. And then, many years later – keeping his promise. Sandy "The Best" Sarza, my go to editor – and one of my closest friends on the planet. She is always the first to read everything I write and as such, she is always the first to ask... "What are you trying to say?" I am never quite sure. Lori Shibinette, who's friendship, insight and support – during some of my most challenging moments, cannot be overstated. Finally, Mistress Kerry Winger. There are some people in your life that make such a huge impact, in so many different areas, that it is hard to point at just one thing and say "That's it," that is why you are so special to me. Mistress Kerry is this person. She is, quite literally, amazing to all who know her and I am privileged to call her my friend.

I wouldn't be anywhere without Mommsie, who's love and support reminds me how I should parent and Kyle Peterson, still the reason I get up so early and work so hard.

A few editorial credits: Did I tell you I have the most amazing friends? Adam Duke, Sandy Sarza, Lori Shibinette, DeAnn Walters and Kerry Winger, all took the time to not only read my manuscript, armed with red pens and yellow highlighters, but then spent (literally) hours on the phone with me. I could not have done it without you and I appreciate every single one of you for your thoughtful insights, analysis and opinions.

Books Cited

Atkins, Robert C. *Dr Atkins' New Diet Revolution.* New York: Avon, 2002. Print.

Beck, Craig. "Fat Guy Friday Weight Loss Secrets Of A Former Fatty." *England:* Viral Success Limited, 2013. Print.

Diaz, Cameron, and Sandra Bark. *The Body Book: The Law of Hunger, the Science of Strength, and Other Ways to Love Your Amazing Body.* New York, NY: HarperWave, An Imprint of HarperCollins, 2015. Print.

Elrod, Hal. *The Miracle Morning: The Not-So-Obvious Secret Guaranteed to Transform Your Life (Before 8AM).* Hal Elrod International, Inc. 2012. Print

Siebold, Steve. *Die Fat or Get Tough: 101 Differences in Thinking between Fat People and Fit People.* England: London House, 2009. Print.